Protecting
THOSE WHO SERVE

*Strategies to Protect the Health of
Deployed U.S. Forces*

Committee on Strategies to Protect the Health of
Deployed U.S. Forces

INSTITUTE OF MEDICINE

NATIONAL ACADEMY PRESS
Washington, D.C.

NATIONAL ACADEMY PRESS • 2101 Constitution Avenue, N.W. • Washington, DC 20418

NOTICE: The project that is the subject of this report was approved by the Governing Board of the National Research Council, whose members are drawn from the councils of the National Academy of Sciences, the National Academy of Engineering, and the Institute of Medicine. The members of the committee responsible for the report were chosen for their special competences and with regard for appropriate balance.

Support for this project was provided by Contract No. DASW01-97-C-0078 between the National Academy of Sciences and the U.S. Department of Defense. The views presented in this report are those of the Institute of Medicine Committee on Strategies to Protect the Health of Deployed U.S. Forces and are not necessarily those of the funding agency.

International Standard Book No. 0-309-07189-5

Additional copies of this report are available for sale from the National Academy Press, 2101 Constitution Avenue, N.W., Box 285, Washington, DC 20055. Call (800) 624-6242 or (202) 334-3313 (in the Washington metropolitan area), or visit the NAP's home page at **www.nap.edu**. The full text of this report is available at **www.nap.edu**.

For more information about the Institute of Medicine, visit the IOM home page at **www.iom.edu**.

Copyright 2000 by the National Academy of Sciences. All rights reserved.

Printed in the United States of America.

The serpent has been a symbol of long life, healing, and knowledge among almost all cultures and religions since the beginning of recorded history. The serpent adopted as a logotype by the Institute of Medicine is a relief carving from ancient Greece, now held by the Staatliche Museen in Berlin.

*"Knowing is not enough; we must apply.
Willing is not enough; we must do."*
—Goethe

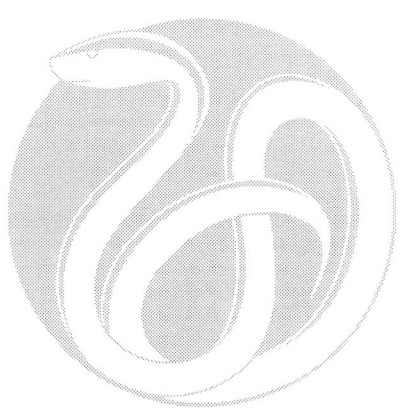

INSTITUTE OF MEDICINE

Shaping the Future for Health

THE NATIONAL ACADEMIES

National Academy of Sciences
National Academy of Engineering
Institute of Medicine
National Research Council

The **National Academy of Sciences** is a private, nonprofit, self-perpetuating society of distinguished scholars engaged in scientific and engineering research, dedicated to the furtherance of science and technology and to their use for the general welfare. Upon the authority of the charter granted to it by the Congress in 1863, the Academy has a mandate that requires it to advise the federal government on scientific and technical matters. Dr. Bruce M. Alberts is president of the National Academy of Sciences.

The **National Academy of Engineering** was established in 1964, under the charter of the National Academy of Sciences, as a parallel organization of outstanding engineers. It is autonomous in its administration and in the selection of its members, sharing with the National Academy of Sciences the responsibility for advising the federal government. The National Academy of Engineering also sponsors engineering programs aimed at meeting national needs, encourages education and research, and recognizes the superior achievements of engineers. Dr. William A. Wulf is president of the National Academy of Engineering.

The **Institute of Medicine** was established in 1970 by the National Academy of Sciences to secure the services of eminent members of appropriate professions in the examination of policy matters pertaining to the health of the public. The Institute acts under the responsibility given to the National Academy of Sciences by its congressional charter to be an adviser to the federal government and, upon its own initiative, to identify issues of medical care, research, and education. Dr. Kenneth I. Shine is president of the Institute of Medicine.

The **National Research Council** was organized by the National Academy of Sciences in 1916 to associate the broad community of science and technology with the Academy's purposes of furthering knowledge and advising the federal government. Functioning in accordance with general policies determined by the Academy, the Council has become the principal operating agency of both the National Academy of Sciences and the National Academy of Engineering in providing services to the government, the public, and the scientific and engineering communities. The Council is administered jointly by both Academies and the Institute of Medicine. Dr. Bruce M. Alberts and Dr. William A. Wulf are chairman and vice chairman, respectively, of the National Research Council.

COMMITTEE ON STRATEGIES TO PROTECT THE HEALTH OF DEPLOYED U.S. FORCES

JOHN H. MOXLEY (*Chair*), Managing Director, North American Health Care Division, Korn/Ferry International, Los Angeles
RUTH L. BERKELMAN, Senior Adviser to the Director, Centers for Disease Control and Prevention, and Rollins School of Public Health, Emory University
J. CRIS BISGARD, Director, Health Services, Delta Air Lines, Atlanta
GUY A. LABOA, Executive Director, Dailies Manufacturing, CIBA Vision, Duluth, Georgia
LAYTON McCURDY, Dean and Vice President of Medical Affairs, Medical University of South Carolina
MATTHEW L. PUGLISI, Government Relations Manager, Optical Society of America, Washington, D.C.
LYNN A. STREETER, Consultant, Knowledge Analysis Technologies, LLC, Boulder, Colorado
ELAINE VAUGHAN, Associate Professor, Department of Psychology and Social Behavior, University of California at Irvine
LAUREN ZEISE, Chief, Reproductive and Cancer Hazard Assessment Section, California Environmental Protection Agency, Oakland

Staff

JOSEPH CASSELLS, Study Director
LOIS JOELLENBECK, Senior Program Officer
PHILLIP BAILEY, Project Assistant
RYAN CATTEAU, Project Assistant
RICHARD MILLER, Director, Medical Follow-Up Agency

REVIEWERS

The report was reviewed by individuals chosen for their diverse perspectives and technical expertise in accordance with procedures approved by the National Research Council's Report Review Committee. The purpose of this independent review is to provide candid and critical comments to assist the authors and the Institute of Medicine in making the published report as sound as possible and to ensure that the report meets institutional standards for objectivity, evidence, and responsiveness to the study charge. The contents of the review comments and the draft manuscript remain confidential to protect the integrity of the deliberative process. The committee wishes to thank the following individuals for their participation in the report review process:

Elizabeth L. Anderson, President and Chief Executive Officer, Sciences International, Inc., Alexandria, Virginia
George Anderson, President, American College of Preventive Medicine, Vienna, Virginia
John C. Bailar III, Professor, Department of Health Studies, The University of Chicago
Paul E. Busick, President and Executive Director, North Carolina Global TransPark Authority, Kinston, North Carolina
Daniel J. Clauw, Associate Professor of Medicine and Othorpedics and Scientific Director, Georgetown Chronic Pain and Fatigue Research Center, and Chief, Division of Rheumatology, Immunology, and Allergy, Georgetown University Medical Center
Paul D. Clayton, Medical Informaticist, Salt Lake City, Utah
Gerald P. Dinneen, Vice President, S&T, Honeywell, Inc., ret., Edina, Minnesota
James Terry Scott, Director, National Security Program, John F. Kennedy School of Government, Harvard University
Harrison Shull, Professor Emeritus, U.S. Naval Postgraduate School, Monterey, California
Stephen B. Thacker, Acting Director, National Center for Injury Prevention and Control, Atlanta

While the individuals listed above provided many constructive comments and suggestions, responsibility for the final content of the report rests solely with the authoring committee and the Institute of Medicine.

Acronyms

AFMIC	Armed Forces Medical Intelligence Center
CBT	cognitive behavior therapy
CDC	Centers for Disease Control and Prevention
CPR	computer-based patient record
DoD	U.S. Department of Defense
HEAR	Health Evaluation and Assessment Review
ICD-9	*International Classification of Diseases,* version 9
IOM	Institute of Medicine
JCS	Joint Chiefs of Staff
NIH	National Institutes of Health
NSTC	National Science and Technology Council
RAP	Recruit Assessment Program
VA	U.S. Department of Veterans Affairs

Contents

EXECUTIVE SUMMARY 1

1 THE PROBLEM 9

2 THE STRATEGY 13
Strategy 1, 14
Strategy 2, 19
Strategy 3, 25
Strategy 4, 29
Strategy 5, 32
Strategy 6, 35

REFERENCES 39

APPENDIXES
A   Study Scope and Statement of Task, 43
B   Strategies to Protect the Health of Deployed U.S. Forces: Analytical Framework for Assessing Risks—Executive Summary, 45
C   Strategies to Protect the Health of Deployed U.S. Forces: Detecting, Characterizing, and Documenting Exposures—Executive Summary, 54
D   Strategies to Protect the Health of Deployed U.S. Forces: Force Protection and Decontamination—Executive Summary, 69

E Strategies to Protect the Health of Deployed U.S. Forces: Medical Surveillance, Record Keeping, and Risk Reduction—Executive Summary, 83
F Acknowledgments, 97
G Committee Biographies, 100

Executive Summary

The 670,000 service members deployed in 1990–1991 to Southwest Asia for Operations Desert Shield and Desert Storm (the Gulf War) were different from the troops deployed in previous similar operations: they were more ethnically diverse, there were more women and more parents, and more activated members of the Reserves and National Guard were uprooted from civilian jobs. The overwhelming victory that they achieved in the Gulf War has been shadowed by subsequent concerns about the long-term health status of those who served. Various constituencies, including a significant number of veterans, speculate that unidentified risk factors led to chronic, medically unexplained illnesses, and these constituencies challenge the depth of the military's commitment to protect the health of deployed troops.

Recognizing the seriousness of these concerns, the U.S. Department of Defense (DoD) has sought assistance over the past decade from numerous expert panels to examine these issues (DoD, 1994; National Institutes of Health Technology Workshop Panel, 1994; IOM, 1996a,b, 1997; Presidential Advisory Committee on Gulf War Veterans' Illnesses, 1996). Although DoD has generally concurred in the findings of these committees, few concrete changes have been made at the field level. The most important recommendations remain unimplemented, despite the compelling rationale for urgent action. A Presidential Review Directive for the National Science and Technology Council to develop an interagency plan to address health preparedness for future deployments led to a 1998 report titled *A National Obligation* (National Science and Technology Council, 1998). Like earlier reports, it outlines a comprehensive program that can be used to meet that obligation, but there has been little progress toward implementation of the program. Recently, the Medical Readiness Division, J-4, of the Joint Staff released a capstone document, *Force Health Protection*, which also describes a commendable vision for protecting deploying forces (The Joint Staff, Medical Readiness Division, 2000). The committee fears that the vision outlined in that report will meet the same fate as the other reports.

With the 10th anniversary of the Gulf War now here, the Committee on Strategies to Protect the Health of Deployed U.S. Forces has concluded that the implementation of the expert panels' recommendations and government-developed plans has been unacceptable. For example, medical encounters in theater are still not necessarily recorded in individuals' medical records, and the locations of service members during deployments are still not documented or archived for future use. In addition, environmental and medical hazards are not yet well integrated in the information provided to commanders. The committee believes that a major reason for this lack of progress is the fact that no single authority within DoD has been assigned responsibility for the implementation of the recommendations and plans. The committee believes, because of the complexity of the tasks involved and the overlapping areas of responsibility involved, that the single authority must rest with the Secretary of Defense.

The committee was charged with advising DoD on a strategy to protect the health of deployed U.S. forces. The committee has concluded that immediate action must be taken to accelerate implementation of these plans to demonstrate the importance that should be placed on protecting the health and well-being of service members. This report describes the challenges and recommends a strategy to better protect the health of deployed forces in the future. Many of the recommendations are restatements of recommendations that have been made before, recommendations that have not been implemented. Further delay could result in unnecessary risks to service members and could jeopardize the accomplishment of future missions. The committee recognizes the critical importance of integrated health risk assessment, improved medical surveillance, accurate troop location information, and exposure monitoring to force health protection. Failure to move briskly on these fronts will further erode the traditional trust between the service member and the leadership.

The four reports completed from the work of the first 2 years of this study (IOM, 1999; NRC, 2000a,c,d) provide detailed discussions and recommendations about areas in which actions are needed to protect the health of deployed forces. The committee has been informed by those reports and endorses the recommendations within them. In the present report, the committee describes six major strategies that address the areas identified from the earlier reports that demand further emphasis and require greater effort by DoD. The committee selected these strategies on the basis of the contents of the four reports, briefings by the principal investigators of those reports, and input from members of the military and other experts in response to the four reports.

- Strategy 1. Use a systematic process to prospectively evaluate non-battle-related risks associated with the activities and settings of deployments.

EXECUTIVE SUMMARY

- Strategy 2. Collect and manage environmental data and personnel location, biological samples, and activity data to facilitate analysis of deployment exposures and to support clinical care and public health activities.
- Strategy 3. Develop the risk assessment, risk management, and risk communication skills of military leaders at all levels.
- Strategy 4. Accelerate implementation of a health surveillance system that spans the service life cycle and that continues after separation from service.
- Strategy 5. Implement strategies to address medically unexplained symptoms in populations that have deployed.
- Strategy 6. Implement a joint computerized patient record and other automated record keeping that meets the information needs of those involved with individual care and military public health.

In the following sections and in the full report that follows this summary the committee outlines recommendations relating to each of these important strategies.

STRATEGY 1

Use a systematic process to prospectively evaluate non-battle-related risks associated with the activities and settings of deployments.

Recommendations

1.1 DoD should designate clear responsibility and accountability for a health risk assessment process encompassing non-battle-related risks and risks from chemical and biological warfare agents as well as traditional battle risks.

- **The multidisciplinary process should include inventorying exposures associated with all aspects of the anticipated activities and settings of deployments.**
- **Commanders should be provided with distillations of integrated health risk assessments that have included consideration of toxic industrial chemicals and long-term effects from low-level exposures.**
- **Service member perceptions and concerns should be factored into the process of risk assessment. This will require assessing common concerns of the affected populations and evaluating whether the contents of risk assessments address those issues critical to cultivating effective risk management and trust in the process.**

1.2 Incidents involving toxic industrial chemicals should be among the scenarios used for military training exercises and war

games to raise awareness of these threats and refine the responses to them.

1.3 DoD should provide additional resources to improve medical and environmental intelligence gathering, analysis, and dissemination to risk assessors and to preventive medicine practitioners. DoD should provide a mechanism for information feedback from the medical community to the medical intelligence system.

1.4 DoD should ensure that medical intelligence is incorporated into the intelligence annex to the operations plan and is considered in shaping the operational plan.

1.5 DoD should devise mechanisms to ensure that state-of-the-art medical knowledge is brought to bear in developing medical annexes to the operational plans and preventive medicine requirements, drawing on expertise both inside and outside DoD.

1.6 DoD should adopt an exposure minimization orientation in which predeployment intelligence about industrial and other environmental hazards is factored into operational plans.

STRATEGY 2

Collect and manage environmental data and personnel location, biological samples, and activity data to facilitate analysis of deployment exposures and to support clinical care and public health activities.

Recommendations

2.1 DoD should assign single responsibility for collecting, managing, and integrating information on non-battle-related hazards.

2.2 DoD should integrate expertise in the nuclear, biological, chemical, and environmental sciences for efficient environmental monitoring of chemical warfare agents and toxic industrial chemicals for both short- and long-term risks.

2.3 For major deployments and deployments in which there is an anticipated threat of chemical exposures, during deployments DoD should collect biological samples such as blood and urine from a sample of deployed forces. Samples can be stored until needed to test for validated biomarkers for possible deployment exposures or analyzed in near real time as needed for high-risk groups.

2.4 DoD should clearly define the individuals permitted access to and the uses of biological samples and the information derived from them. DoD should communicate these policies to the service members and establish a process to review ethical issues related to operational data collection and use.

2.5 DoD should ensure that adequate preventive medicine assets including laboratory capability are available to analyze deployment exposure data in near real time and respond appropriately.

2.6 DoD should ensure that the deployed medical contingent from command surgeons to unit medics has mission-essential information on the likely non-battle-related hazards of the deployments and access to timely updates.

2.7 DoD should implement a joint system for recording, archiving, and retrieving information on the locations of service member units during operations.

2.8 Environmental monitoring, biomarker, and troop location and activity databases should all be designed to permit linkages with one another and with individual medical records. It is crucial that means be developed to link environmental data to individual records.

STRATEGY 3

Develop the risk assessment, risk management, and risk communication skills of military leaders at all levels.

Recommendations

3.1 DoD should provide training in the contemporary principles of health risk assessment and health risk management to leaders at all levels to convey understanding of the capabilities and uncertainties in these processes.

3.2 DoD should institutionalize training in risk communication for commanders and health care providers. Periodic formal evaluation and monitoring of the quality of training programs should be standard procedure. Risk communication should be framed as a dynamic process that is responsive to input from several sources, changing concerns of affected populations, modifications in scientific risk evidence, and newly identified needs for communication.

3.3 DoD should jump start training in risk communication by delivering it at appropriate settings for various levels of service, including at the time of initial entry into service and at the service schools. DoD should give particular attention to the training of medical officers on initial entry into service. Opportunities for supplemental training and support of ongoing education in risk communication should be formally identified.

3.4 DoD should include the stakeholders (service members, their families, and community representatives) in the development of a plan for DoD risk communication to include when and how risk communications should take place when new concerns arise.

STRATEGY 4

Accelerate implementation of a health surveillance system that spans the service life cycle and that continues after separation from service.

Recommendations

4.1 DoD should establish clear leadership authority and accountability to coordinate preventive medicine—including environmental and health surveillance, training, and investigation—within and across the individual services and DoD. DoD should ensure that adequate preventive medicine personnel and resources are available early on deployments.

4.2 DoD should collect health status and risk factor data on recruits as they enter the military, as planned through the Recruit Assessment Program, now in the pilot stage. DoD should maintain health status data for both active-duty and reserve service members with annual health surveys.

4.3 DoD should continue to collect self-reported health information from service members after their deployments to permit comparisons with their predeployment health and with the health of other service members. For a representative sample of those who leave the military health system, DoD should continue to administer the annual health status survey for 2 to 5 years after a major deployment to learn about health changes after deployments.

4.4 DoD should mandate central reporting of notifiable conditions including laboratory findings across the services. DoD should strengthen public health laboratory capabilities and integrate laboratory and epidemiological resources to facilitate appropriate analysis and investigation.

STRATEGY 5

Implement strategies to address medically unexplained symptoms in populations that have been deployed.

Recommendations

5.1 DoD should include information about medically unexplained symptoms in the training and risk communication information for service members at all levels.

5.2 DoD should complete and implement guidelines for the management of patients with medically unexplained symptoms in the military health system. DoD should provide primary health care and other health care providers with training about medically unexplained symptoms and in the use of the guidelines. DoD should carry out clinical trials to accompany the implementation of the guidelines and evaluate their impact.

5.3 DoD should establish a treatment outcomes and health services research program within DoD to further provide an empirical basis for improvement of treatment programs to address medically unexplained symptoms. This program should be carried out in collaboration and cooperation with the U.S. Department of Veterans Affairs health system and the U.S. Department of Health and Human Services.

5.4 DoD should design and implement a research plan to better understand predisposing, precipitating, and perpetuating factors for medically unexplained symptoms in military populations.

STRATEGY 6

Implement a joint computerized patient record and other automated record keeping that meets the information needs of those involved with individual care and military public health.

Recommendations

6.1 DoD should treat the development of a lifetime computer-based patient record for service members as a major acquisition, with commensurate high-level responsibility, accountability, and coordination. Clear goals, strategies, implementation plans, milestones, and costs must be defined and approved with input from the end users.

6.2 DoD should accelerate development and implementation of automated systems to gather mission-critical data elements. DoD should deploy a system that fills the basic needs of the military mission first but is consistent with the architecture and data standards planned for the overall system.

6.3 DoD should implement the electronic data system to allow the transfer of data between DoD and the U.S. Department of Veterans Affairs.

6.4 DoD should establish an external advisory board that reports to the Secretary of Defense to provide ongoing review and advice regarding the military health information system's strategy and implementation.

6.5 DoD should include immunization data, ambulatory care data, and data from deployment exposures with immediate medical implications in the individual medical records and should develop a mechanism for linking individual records to other databases with information about deployment exposures.

6.6 DoD should develop methods to gather and analyze retrievable, electronically stored health data on reservists. At a minimum, DoD should establish records of military immunizations for all reservists. DoD should work toward a computerized patient record that contains information from the Recruit Assessment Program and periodic health assessments and develop such records first for those most likely to deploy early.

1

The Problem

The 670,000 service members deployed in 1990–1991 to Southwest Asia for Operations Desert Shield and Desert Storm (the Gulf War) were different from the troops deployed in previous similar operations: they were more ethnically diverse, there were more women and more parents, and more activated members of the Reserves and National Guard were uprooted from civilian jobs. The overwhelming victory that they achieved in the Gulf War has been shadowed by subsequent concerns about the long-term health status of those who served. Various constituencies, including a significant number of veterans, speculate that unidentified risk factors led to chronic, medically unexplained illnesses, and these constituencies challenge the depth of the military's commitment to protect the health of deployed troops.

Recognizing the seriousness of these concerns, the U.S. Department of Defense (DoD) has sought assistance over the past decade from numerous expert panels to examine these issues (DoD, 1994; National Institute of Health Technology Workshop Panel, 1994; IOM, 1996a,b, 1997; Presidential Advisory Committee on Gulf War Veterans' Illnesses, 1996). Although DoD has generally concurred in the findings of these committees, few concrete changes have been made at the field level. The most important recommendations remain unimplemented, despite the compelling rationale for urgent action. A Presidential Review Directive for the National Science and Technology Council to develop an interagency plan to address health preparedness for future deployments led to a 1998 report titled *A National Obligation* (National Science and Technology Council, 1998). Like earlier reports, it outlines a comprehensive program that can be used to meet that obligation, but there has been little progress toward implementation of the program. Recently, the Medical Readiness Division, J-4, of the Joint Staff released a capstone document, *Force Health Protection*, which also describes a commendable vision for protecting deploying forces (The Joint Staff, Medical Readiness Division, 2000). The committee fears that the vision outlined in that report will meet the same fate as the other reports.

With the 10th anniversary of the Persian Gulf War now here, the Committee on Strategies to Protect the Health of Deployed U.S. Forces has concluded that the implementation of the expert panels' recommendations and government-developed plans has been unacceptable. For example, medical encounters in theater are still not necessarily recorded in individuals' medical records, and the locations of service members during deployments are still not documented or archived for future use. In addition, environmental and medical hazards are not yet well integrated in the information provided to commanders. The committee believes that a major reason for this lack of progress is the fact that no single authority within DoD has been assigned responsibility for the implementation of the recommendations and plans. The committee believes, because of the complexity of the tasks involved and the overlapping areas of responsibility involved, that the single authority must rest with the Secretary of Defense.

The committee has concluded that immediate action must be taken to accelerate implementation of these plans to demonstrate the importance that should be placed on protecting the health and well-being of service members. This report describes the challenges and recommends a strategy to better protect the health of deployed forces in the future. Many of the recommendations are restatements of recommendations that have been made before, recommendations that have not been implemented. Further delay could result in unnecessary risks to service members and could jeopardize the accomplishment of future missions. The committee recognizes the critical importance of integrated health risk assessment, improved medical surveillance, accurate troop location information, and exposure monitoring to force health protection. Failure to move briskly on these fronts will further erode the traditional trust between the service member and the leadership.

In recent years, U.S. service members have frequently deployed to smaller-scale contingency operations, including operations that involve humanitarian assistance, disaster relief, peacekeeping, enforcement of sanctions, arms control, counterterrorism, counter-drug action, and counter-insurgencies, with the range of combat risk being from low to high (Reuter, 1999). The potential settings of deployments have multiplied along with the types of operations that might be required. Many different climates and terrains are possible and must be factored into the consideration of potential deployment scenarios. The challenges posed by rapidly expanding technologies and interaction with coalition partners during deployments also must be met. This changing environment requires DoD to respond in less traditional ways and has greatly influenced the preparation of this report.

As of the end of February 2000, more than 40,000 U.S. personnel—active-duty, reserves, and civilian employees—were deployed to 15 operations. The largest number in a single deployment was nearly 16,000 participants in Operation Southern Watch, whereas some of the smaller operations had as few as 10 deployed personnel (LTC G. Harper, Personnel Readiness Division, Joint Chiefs of Staff, personal communication, March 2, 2000).

This increased deployment schedule and the increased mobilization of reserve personnel to support these deployments may contribute to problems with recruitment and retention. The Army fell 6,290 individuals short of its goal of 74,500 new recruits in fiscal year 1999. During fiscal year 2000, the Army's goal is to enlist 80,000 active-duty individuals (Army News Service, 1999). Trust in DoD leadership will be enhanced when political leaders and military commanders communicate to the general public a clear rationale for any future deployments, particularly in operations other than war, coupled with a sincere commitment to the health and well-being of affected service members.

The events that followed the conclusion of the Gulf War are instructive. Despite the different makeup of the force and the low casualty rate, national leaders, remembering Vietnam, did anticipate some postconflict health concerns and initiated programs to address them. The programs were chiefly focused on helping veterans readjust to civilian life and cope with the aftermath of war.

However, shortly after returning from the Gulf, some men and women began to experience debilitating illnesses and complained that they were not being taken seriously by physicians in DoD and the U.S. Department of Veterans Affairs (VA). As the number of these veterans increased, first VA and later DoD established registries to identify and treat these veterans' illnesses. Although the majority of these veterans had readily diagnosed illnesses, for a significant number of veterans their illnesses remained medically unexplained, which led to much speculation about the possible relationship of their illnesses with various risk factors, other than combat, that were present in the Gulf (Presidential Advisory Committee on Gulf War Veterans' Illnesses, 1996). Several expert committees were asked to examine those various risk factors and to determine whether a "unique" Gulf War illness with a known cause could be established (DoD, 1994; National Institutes of Health Technology Workshop Panel, 1994; IOM, 1996a,b; Presidential Advisory Committee on Gulf War Veterans' Illnesses, 1996). Each of these panels concluded that there was no evidence consistent with the existence of a unique illness and that no single cause could be established. That remains the case, despite a vigorous research portfolio examining multiple hypotheses put forward as possible explanations for the medically unexplained physical symptoms experienced by these sick veterans. This continuing controversy highlights, in a very visible way, the tensions that exist between expectations and realities, between science and politics, and between policy and execution.

In the summer of 1996 Deputy Secretary of Defense John White met with the leadership of the National Research Council and the Institute of Medicine to explore the idea of a proactive effort to learn from lessons of the Gulf War and other deployments (e.g., those to Somalia, Haiti, and Bosnia) and to develop a strategy to better protect the health of U.S. troops in future deployments. DoD sought an external, independent, and unbiased evaluation of its efforts regarding the protection of U.S. forces in four areas: (1) assessment of health risks during deployments in hostile environments, (2) technologies and methods for detection and tracking of exposures to a subset of harmful agents, (3) physical protection and decontamination, and (4) medical protection, health consequences and treatment, and medical record keeping. Particular emphasis was to be placed on chemical and biological warfare injuries and disease and non-battle injuries from chemical contaminants in the environment. These studies were conducted concurrently by the Commission on Life Sciences, Commission on Engineering and Technical Systems, and the Institute of Medicine, all components of the National Research Council. The four technical reports and a workshop summary prepared by these units were completed in the fall of 1999 (IOM, 1999; NRC, 2000a–d). These reports were circulated to various divisions, services, and agencies within DoD with responsibilities in these technical areas. Comments were received in writing and in person.

In the study's final year, the present Institute of Medicine committee was formed and used those responses and the reports developed by the four respective sets of principal investigators and advisory panels as a starting point to inform this final report (the executive summary of each technical report is included in Appendixes B to E of this report; the statement of task is found in Appendix A). The committee believes that these technical reports can stand on their own merits and endorses the recommendations that they contain. It has not been the present committee's intent to recapitulate or summarize those reports. Rather, the committee used them to extend the findings and recommendations that it considered to be most important to a long-term strategy for protection of the health of deployed forces, and to expand on broader, cross-cutting issues. The committee urges deliberate action to bring about concrete changes in response to recommendations in those reports.

The committee's overriding concern is that everything consistent with mission accomplishment be done to protect the health and lives of U.S. service members who are knowingly placed in harm's way. The committee understands that the changes will be costly and will inflict the pain of organizational change. The Department of Defense, however, has the obligation to avoid unnecessary disease, injury, disability, and death as it pursues the accomplishment of its missions. Not to fulfill that obligation would be simply unconscionable.

2

The Strategy

The four reports completed from the work of the first 2 years of this study (IOM, 1999; NRC 2000a,c,d) provide detailed discussions and recommendations about areas in which actions are needed to protect the health of deployed forces. The Committee on Strategies to Protect the Health of Deployed U.S. Forces has been informed by those reports and endorses the recommendations within them. In the present report the committee describes six major strategies that address areas identified from the earlier reports that demand further emphasis and require greater effort by the U.S. Department of Defense (DoD). The committee selected these strategies on the basis of the contents of the four reports, briefings by the principal investigators of those reports, and input from members of the military and other experts in response to the four reports.

- Strategy 1. Use a systematic process to prospectively evaluate non-battle-related risks associated with the activities and settings of deployments.
- Strategy 2. Collect and manage environmental data and personnel location, biological samples, and activity data to facilitate analysis of deployment exposures and to support clinical care and public health activities.
- Strategy 3. Develop the risk assessment, risk management, and risk communication skills of military leaders at all levels.
- Strategy 4. Accelerate implementation of a health surveillance system that spans the service life cycle and that continues after separation from service.
- Strategy 5. Implement strategies to address medically unexplained symptoms in populations that have deployed.

- Strategy 6. Implement a joint computerized patient record and other automated record keeping that meets the information needs of those involved with individual care and military public health.

In the report that follows, the committee outlines recommendations relating to each of these important strategies.

STRATEGY 1

Use a systematic process to prospectively evaluate non-battle-related risks associated with the activities and settings of deployments.[1]

Managing risk is a complex task that requires a strong partnership between the parties involved. Health risk assessment is a tool that can aid decision making and strengthen the military enterprise[2]. The process of risk evaluation performs optimally when it provides a comprehensive profile of the primary agents and activities that may affect the health of deployed troops, promotes reasoned choices by commanders and military planners, and is responsive to the legitimate questions of service members and their families. DoD and the military services have made progress in the programs and processes that they use to assess deployment-related health risks to service members. However, significant work is needed for better integration of the information gathered and for more effective conveyance of that information to decision makers. Particular challenges exist in assessing and integrating the risks from environmental chemicals, chemical and biological warfare agents, and the array of disease and non-battle injury risks to deployed forces. In this section, the committee describes additional initiatives required from DoD to assess deployment-related health risks and provide integrated information about these risks to commanders and medical personnel.

A systematic process is needed for evaluation of deployment-related health risks. This process should take into account not only potentially hazardous agents but also the likely steps and actions within a deployment that could expose service members to health risks. The methods could be similar to those used in pollution prevention efforts in both civilian and military settings, which involve review of the life cycle of hypothetical deployments to consider the ac-

---

[1] In the first 2 years of the National Research Council-Institute of Medicine Strategies to Protect the Health of Deployed U.S. Forces project, Lorenz Rhomberg carried out a study charged with developing an analytical framework for assessing the risks to the health of deployed forces, particularly from disease and non-battle-related injuries or from chemical or biological warfare agents. The National Research Council report *Strategies to Protect the Health of Deployed U.S. Forces: Analytical Framework for Assessing Risks* (NRC, 2000a,b) describes the framework and is the starting point for this section. The executive summary of that report is found in Appendix B.

[2] Health risk assessment includes consideration of both health endpoints and exposure assessment.

tivities that occur, the exposures entailed, the materials consumed, the wastes produced, and the accidents and failures that might occur. The reviews would take into account the range of different missions and settings to which service members may be deployed. Although the committee understands that implementation of the full range of prevention measures or controls may not be possible in settings with high levels of combat-related risks to life and limb, a thorough inventory of possible risks that might be encountered in the course of deployment activities can help in planning and prioritization. The practice of reviewing activities in their entirety and likely settings should prompt consideration of what might be hazardous and what further investigation is needed to understand their safety and risks. Information on all non-battle-related risks should be provided to commanders in an integrated form so that they are readily considered together in the context of all risks to service members.

Part of the challenge for the integrated analysis of deployment activities needed is the fragmentation of health and safety expertise found in both civilian and military settings. Different organizations and groups of people within them are responsible for assessing the risks from infectious diseases, industrial chemicals, equipment, and the array of battle injury threats, including chemical and biological warfare agents. Yet, any given activity within a deployment could contain risks from bullets, climate, chemicals, noise, lasers, infectious diseases, psychological stress, and so forth, in many possible combinations. A systematic evaluation of deployment activities to identify deployment hazards will therefore require overcoming institutional barriers to provide interdisciplinary consideration of these hazards. **As deployment circumstances become increasingly varied, the multidisciplinary perspective is even more essential for accurate assessment of the different elements of risk that may arise.**

When deployments are considered in their entirety, assessing risks from combinations of agents and activities poses an additional challenge. Different exposures can interact additively, synergistically, or antagonistically, raising many questions about potential health risks. Unfortunately, little guidance is available in the civilian sector on how to assess potential synergism among mixtures of risks that include biological agents, chemical agents, physical and other environmental processes (e.g., climate conditions), and psychological stress. Continued research is needed to begin to sort out a hierarchy of potential hazards from such combinations. In the meantime the military should continue to pursue strategies of minimization of exposure to agents that might cause significant short-term effects as well as those that might cause long-term or delayed health effects. Such an exposure minimization orientation is one in which, in the absence of complete information about the health risks posed by particular compounds, efforts are made to use them with caution and limit exposure to them.

Uncertainty is an inevitable component of health risk assessment. It can be reduced with careful efforts to consider activities in their entirety, but uncertainty will remain because of the still-limited knowledge of all aspects of exposures and health effects, and this uncertainty must be conveyed to decision makers.

Although for decades organizations within the military have been dedicated to assessing risks from chemical warfare agents and infectious diseases, consideration of the array of other potentially hazardous chemicals that might be encountered is more recent. Because of the enormous array of industrial chemicals in use around the world, it is a tremendous challenge to evaluate the risks they pose, particularly at low levels. It is also difficult to measure human exposure at low levels. Despite its difficulty, however, this challenge should not be ignored. Efforts have begun to include assessment of the risks from toxic industrial chemicals in military planning and risk assessment activities, but **continued effort is needed to integrate consideration of both the acute effects of exposure to these chemicals and the risks posed by long-term, low-level exposures.**[3] The assessment results must be integrated into the spectrum of potential hazards accounted for before and during deployments. The potential long-term effects of other exposures during deployments must also be part of the assessment of risks from deployment activities. This integrated health risk assessment will therefore be complex and detailed in its entirety, but should be summarized in a chart or matrix to be provided to the commander for decision making. The additional resources required for this challenging task must be identified and developed. Furthermore, the risk management concepts derived from these efforts should be included in scenarios used for military exercises and war games, with the lessons learned used to further refine the assessment and planning process.

Contemporary models of health risk management and assessment suggest that effective responses to risk situations require a broad understanding of the values of importance to the affected populations (Fisher, 1991; International Life Sciences Institute, 1993; Kasperson and Kasperson, 1996; Kuehn, 1996; Kunreuther and Slovic, 1996; NRC, 1996). Without accommodation of these concerns by the assessment process, analyses may not adequately address the right questions, may increase the perceived uncertainty about an exposure situation, and may undermine the partnerships required to implement plans and policies. **Therefore, a primary objective of the decision-making process is to integrate the values and concerns of affected and interested parties into scientific procedures.** Health risk assessments should thus be the outcome of an analytic and deliberative process—a process that should include early consideration of the problem from several perspectives. Incorporating the concerns of service members will necessitate a review of the questions posed for analysis (e.g., most likely scenario versus worst-case scenario), the data required, and the risk consequences considered (e.g., the long-term health consequences as well as the acute effects of exposure). In risk management situations anticipated to be

---

[3] In the National Research Council report *Strategies to Protect the Health of Deployed U.S. Forces: Detecting, Characterizing, and Documenting Exposures* (NRC, 2000c), principal investigator Thomas McKone describes the need for dose-response information to evaluate the effects of "low-level" exposures. This information is crucial to establishing criteria for detecting and monitoring low-level exposures to chemicals. The executive summary of that report is found in Appendix C.

controversial, it is particularly important that the analytic-deliberative process be inclusive and iterative (NRC, 1996).

In practice, the groups responsible for assessing deployment health risks should involve focus groups to gain some service member input regarding the concerns raised by various aspects of deployment activities. Future assessments should also be informed by past conflicts in which interested parties explicitly detailed key risk and health issues that were perceived to have been ignored in formal assessments and previous decisions. Records of past congressional and expert panel hearings on risk and the health of deployed troops (e.g., Agent Orange in Vietnam and illnesses in Gulf War veterans), as well as other discussions in the public sector regarding community exposures, represent a rich source of information for pending health risk assessments. The organization appointed to carry on the work of the DoD Office of the Special Assistant for Gulf War Illnesses should provide another source of information from lessons that have already been learned. The formal analysis of such material could offer DoD guidance about which dimensions of exposure situations frequently emerge as principal considerations for service members, their families, and diverse lay populations. A substantial body of work also exists in the scientific literature regarding lay populations' evaluations of and perspectives on risk situations (Slovic, 1987; Fischhoff et al., 1993; NRC, 1996). DoD might also consider soliciting experts from academia and other non-military settings for advice about integrating service members' perspectives into the process of risk estimation and assessment.

Review of deployment activities and settings to anticipate threats and health risks requires accurate information from the intelligence community. In addition to intelligence about the military threat, information about the climate, the epidemiology of endemic infectious diseases, the safety of the local blood supply, and the locations, raw materials, and products of nearby industries must be considered to identify potential hazards to deploying service members. This information is considered medical intelligence. Significant improvements in the collection and communication of this information to commanders and the medical community are needed. Improvements in the communication of information from the medical community to the medical intelligence organization are also needed.

As mentioned earlier, toxic industrial chemicals are fairly new to the mix of hazards included in risk assessment and are recent additions to medical intelligence gathering. The Armed Forces Medical Intelligence Center (AFMIC) has evolved from a group in the U.S. Army responsible for gathering information on endemic infectious diseases and health care infrastructures in other countries into a joint, cross-service organization. Recently, it has established an environmental branch that assesses the presence of toxic industrial chemicals in other countries. AFMIC is small, however, a total of only about 40 analysts, and requires additional resources to be effective. The health risk assessment effort should include increased cooperation between AFMIC and the environmental health risk assessment groups at the U.S. Army Center for Health Promotion and Preventive Medicine, the Naval Environmental Health Center, and the Air Force Institute for Environment, Safety, and Occupational Health Risk Analysis.

Communication and coordination between the medical intelligence community and the deployed medical community need to be improved. The preventive medicine officers are those best able to interpret and act on the intelligence gathered, so they need access to this information. Currently, however, medical intelligence information is not available to most deployed preventive medicine professionals because of their lack of access to classified databases and communications, particularly in deployed and remote locations.

Medical intelligence must make its way to the commanders as well as to the medical community. One way to ensure this is to include it in the intelligence annex to the operations plan. The operations plan is written by commanders to anticipate the actions and requirements of a particular deployment, and the intelligence annex is a particularly important aspect of this plan. In the past, medical intelligence information has been included in the medical annex to the operations plan, which tends to come near the end of the document, where it runs the risk of being ignored. Placing it in the intelligence annex will better convey the importance of the information to commanders as well as to medical personnel.

Improvement is also needed in the medical annex and preventive medicine requirements written to provide direction for medical preparations and care during the deployment. The annex should incorporate up-to-date medical and preventive medicine information both from external sources and from resources across DoD.

It is also vital that there be a flow of information from medical personnel and others with access to information at the unit level back to the medical intelligence community to better inform members of the community of future needs. The preventive medicine and other health care personnel (e.g., medical corps personnel) involved with deployments on the ground have access to valuable information about the risks that service members are encountering daily, including unanticipated hazards that are manifested during the operation. Their experiences and observations would enrich the understanding of the operation and its setting to provide valuable lessons for the future. A barrier to this transfer of information has been the fact that the medical and intelligence communities work in very separate spheres. However, mechanisms are already in place to collect and review the lessons learned from deployments within the medical community, and these should also be shared with the medical intelligence group and all services.

Strategy 1 Recommendations

1.1 DoD should designate clear responsibility and accountability for a health risk assessment process encompassing non-battle-related risks and risks from chemical and biological warfare agents as well as traditional battle risks.

- **The multidisciplinary process should include inventorying exposures associated with all aspects of the anticipated activities and settings of deployments.**

THE STRATEGY

- Commanders should be provided with distillations of integrated health risk assessments that have included consideration of toxic industrial chemicals and long-term effects from low-level exposures.
- Service member perceptions and concerns should be factored into the process of risk assessment. This will require assessing common concerns of the affected populations and evaluating whether the contents of risk assessments address those issues critical to cultivating effective risk management and trust in the process.

1.2 Incidents involving toxic industrial chemicals should be among the scenarios used for military training exercises and war games to raise awareness of these threats and refine the responses to them.

1.3 DoD should provide additional resources to improve medical and environmental intelligence gathering, analysis, and dissemination to risk assessors and to preventive medicine practitioners. DoD should provide a mechanism for information feedback from the medical community to the medical intelligence system.

1.4 DoD should ensure that medical intelligence is incorporated into the intelligence annex to the operations plan and is considered in shaping the operational plan.

1.5 DoD should devise mechanisms to ensure that state-of-the-art medical knowledge is brought to bear in developing medical annexes to the operational plans and preventive medicine requirements, drawing on expertise both inside and outside DoD.

1.6 DoD should adopt an exposure minimization orientation in which predeployment intelligence about industrial and other environmental hazards is factored into operational plans.

STRATEGY 2

Collect and manage environmental data and personnel location, biological samples, and activity data to facilitate analysis of deployment exposures and to support clinical care and public health activities.

Service members must be confident that the military is doing its best to protect their health to the greatest extent possible for each mission. In recent years both military populations and society at large have demonstrated increased concern about delayed or long-term effects from environmental exposures as well as from vaccines and other medical prophylactics. DoD and the services must have in place systems that can be used to collect and manage the information necessary to make sound health protection decisions and modify them over time as needed.

Collecting information about the environmental, infectious disease, psychological, and other non-battle-related risks of deployment should be an operational requirement. How much information is it necessary to gather? As discussed for Strategy 1, health risk assessment before deployment can help to identify risks most likely to be associated with the activities of a deployment. On the basis of that health risk assessment, decisions must be made about what environmental data and biological samples might be most useful to collect in the field. The sampling plan may change as additional needs for environmental or biological samples become apparent during the deployment.

Preventive medicine planners should prioritize the collection and analysis of environmental samples on the basis of both the mission, including the planned activities of the troops, and the site of deployment and assessment of threats in the area. Statistical sampling and sample stratification strategies should be developed to the extent possible to help meet needs for data collection[4] (NRC, 2000c). Not every sample collected can or should be analyzed; some (particularly biological materials) could be stored for testing of specific hypotheses as they arise (e.g., Gulf War illnesses and environmental exposures).

There is a danger of collecting so many samples (to carefully characterize a given setting) that the system is bogged down. A minimal data set could be determined on the basis of a decision analysis approach referred to in the previous National Research Council (NRC) report (2000c). This approach views information as a means to improve decision making under uncertainty; information is valuable only if it can affect current or future decision making. The challenge is to determine the minimum amount of information needed to inform decisions related to both immediate and long-term health risks, given that uncertainty is inevitable. For this, a tiered approach to prioritizing data collection based on a dimensions of harm scale could be used (Figure 2-1). The dimensions of harm are measured along three scales: the time to effect, the number of individuals at risk, and the severity of the consequences. Larger numbers of individuals at risk and more severe consequences are of higher priority, as are, often, harms with shorter times to their effects. The most crucial data to be gathered are those about imminent hazards with potentially catastrophic effects, when the data can have an influence on the decisions to be made (GEO-CENTERS, Inc., and Life Systems, Inc., for the U.S. Army Center for Environmental Health Research 1997; NRC, 2000c). Data relating to delayed or chronic effects in large numbers would also be important. However, different deployment scenarios will dictate different

---

[4]This section draws on the work in *Strategies to Protect the Health of Deployed U.S. Forces: Detecting, Characterizing, and Documenting Exposures* (NRC, 2000c).

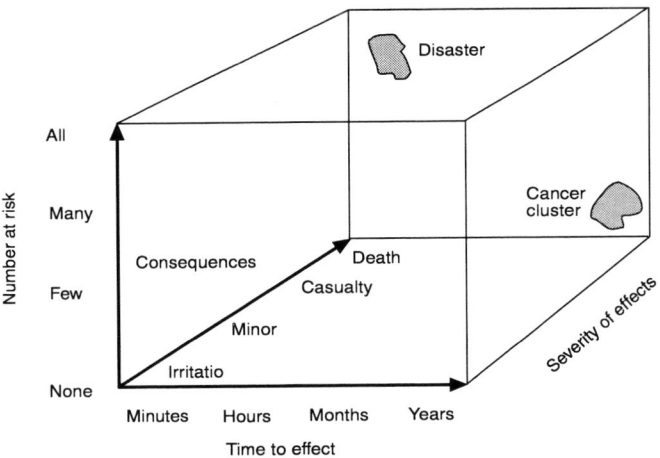

FIGURE 2-1 Dimensions-of-harm scale. SOURCE: GEO-CENTERS, Inc., and Life Systems, Inc., for the U.S. Army Center for Environmental Health Research, 1997.

evaluations of priorities. To the extent possible, the exposure minimization approach applied at garrison in peacetime should carry over to the deployment.

Different information will need to be made available to different parties at different time scales before, during, and after a deployment. The commander will need information in advance about the spectrum of disease and non-battle-related risks facing the troops in a deployment setting so that, together with staff (who will provide integrated engineering, safety, preventive medicine, nuclear, biological, and chemical information), he or she can plan protective and control measures and determine the potential impact of risks and countermeasures on accomplishment of the mission. During the deployment, the commander will need real-time information, with a priority on those risks that affect many people, have a short time to consequences, and that have consequences of death or casualties, that is, that affect accomplishment of the mission. Different deployment scenarios will prompt different evaluations of priorities, and long-term consequences will take on greater import when risks of immediate effects (from bullets, for example) are lower. Health care providers for service members after deployments have other information needs. Health care providers, as well as commanders, service members, and their families, need timely information not just about events with short-term consequences but also about known exposures that may pose future risks to service members and exposures that may pose risks to fewer individuals. Military acquisition personnel will also need information, but they will need this information far in advance of deployments, when they are striving to anticipate the uses and attendant risks of equipment.

Priority setting for collection and archiving of biological samples for potential analysis is also needed, particularly during deployments.[5] Increasingly, the biomedical community has developed the capability to detect chemical or toxic agents and metabolites in biological samples, such as blood, serum, and urine.[6] Markers in other biological samples such as saliva and hair may become increasingly useful for monitoring exposures to a large number of harmful chemicals (NRC, 2000c) as the technology advances. For substances for which such a biomarker has been developed and validated and when a putative exposure has occurred, analysis of biological samples collected from deployed forces may help to assess past exposures. Environmental monitoring is important to allow avoidance or minimization of an exposure before it has occurred. If an exposure may have occurred, biological sampling may be far more efficient than environmental area sampling for the documentation of human exposure. The use of biological samples can be more efficient than the use of environmental area samples in that biological samples can indicate and help to document that human exposure has actually occurred. This permits intervention to prevent further exposures and to give appropriate medical care where needed.

Currently, DoD stores sera collected from all deployed forces within a year before deployment[7] and immediately following certain designated deployments. This practice should continue. Biomonitoring, which currently requires urine or serum for most testing, is not a trivial exercise, especially during a deployment. Sampling may be difficult and interfere with the mission, and the logistics and cost may be quite high for each specimen. Yet, biological samples may also be of great value should unanticipated questions arise later. Thus, during major deployments or deployments with a threat from chemical or industrial agents, biological specimens should be collected from a small subset of individuals, and these samples should be archived for analysis should the need arise. Ideally, these would be drawn as part of a sampling strategy with statistical validity; however, this is frequently not feasible. In such situations a statistical sample should not be required, but samples should be sought in a purposeful manner to maximize useful information about individual exposures. In addition, if the po-

---

[5]This section primarily addresses monitoring for environmental and toxic exposures. However, the committee expects that specimen collection and laboratory testing for infectious diseases for both individual patient needs and detection of epidemics should continue, with adequate infectious disease laboratory capacity assured.

[6]The laboratory of the National Center for Environmental Health of the Centers for Disease Control and Prevention can rapidly screen blood and urine for 90 chemical agents and is anticipated to be able to screen blood and urine for more than 150 chemical agents by September 2001 (National Center for Environmental Health, 2000; James Pirkle, Medical Director, Environmental Health Laboratories, National Center for Environmental Health, personal communication to Ruth Berkelman, May 3, 2000, and June 26, 2000).

[7]Sera are collected for human immunodeficiency virus screens, which are mandatory every 2 years, or within 1 year before a deployment.

tential for an exposure in the field is known to be high or troops develop symptoms potentially indicative of a chemical or infectious exposure, biological samples from potentially exposed troops may be collected in a targeted fashion and tested immediately.

Collection of biological samples from service members that might be stored indefinitely and used for as-yet-undeveloped analyses raises reasonable questions about protections of the confidentiality of such information. Some protections are already in place for the tissue samples collected for remains identification and the serum samples from human immunodeficiency virus testing.[8] It is crucial that safeguards be in place for other types of biological samples to protect the privacy of individuals. Clear statements of the intended uses of data from biological samples should be provided, and guidelines and policies for consideration of subsequent modifications to the intended uses should be developed and made available (IOM, 1999).

Even with the development of biomonitoring, environmental monitoring should continue to be used before and during deployment, as this can permit avoidance of hazardous exposures during deployments. Expertise in both environmental monitoring and biomonitoring is needed so that the fields are integrated noncompetitively and the advances in each field are used most effectively and efficiently to protect the health of the individuals deployed.

It is vital that the locations of units and individuals during deployments be documented, together with activity information. This information is important not only for real-time command decision making on the battlefield but also for enabling the reconstruction of deployment exposures for epidemiological studies and the provision of appropriate medical care after the deployment.[9] However, despite painful lessons learned from both the Vietnam War and Operations Desert Shield and Desert Storm, adequate systems for recording and archiving the locations of deployed forces are still not in place. At present, the tracking of service member locations varies with the deployment. In the current deployment to Kosovo, troops are tracked at the unit level. Each week, the unit provides the task force commander a unit situation report that describes where the unit was located over the previous week. If necessary, these data could be linked with rosters of the individuals in units (collected by the Defense Manpower Data Center) to arrive at an approximation of the locations of individuals for that

---

[8]A series of special rules and procedures protects the privacy interests in the tissue samples collected for identification of remains and any analysis of the DNA from these samples (IOM, 1999). Guidelines on the use of samples from the DoD Serum Repository exist (http://amsa.army.mil), and the repository is subject to "rules and procedures to protect privacy interest of members and ensure exclusive use of specimens for the identification, prevention and control of injuries and diseases associated with military operations" (DoD, 1997, p. 3).

[9]Detailed discussion of tracking the locations and time-activity budgets of deployed military personnel is found in NRC, 2000b, pp. 110–124.

time. Such weekly tracking is not being done for current deployments to Bosnia, Saudi Arabia, and Kuwait.

Information about which units are deployed to a theater of operations and who is present in the units is gathered separately by each service and is transmitted to the DoD Deputy Chief of Staff for Personnel. These data are frequently inaccurate and out of date because no system has been designated for the collection, maintenance, and forwarding of the information from the units. The data also are not available to the preventive medicine community in real time or even within a short period of time after a deployment. Those trying to carry out surveillance must thus work without good denominators.

Miniaturized Global Positioning Satellite technology is now available and is integrated with consumer and military devices, such as cellular telephones. Troops can thus be tracked in real time. However, systems have not been built to capture these location data, catalogue and archive them, or, when security concerns permit the provision of these data, make them available for retrospective analyses and in real time to preventive medicine officers. The committee urges rapid progress toward this goal.

The collection of detailed information about the locations and activities of service members could have costs in terms of privacy and could result in potential misuse of the technology. Careful thought about how such technology could be applied must take into consideration the potential for thwarting the systems (willfully deceiving the system), unnecessarily intruding in private activities, or revealing information to the enemy. Clear explanation of the justification for real-time tracking must be provided during service member training.

Careful coordination is lacking for the planning and execution of data collection activities related to environmental monitoring, biomonitoring, and personnel activity and location information. Data systems must be planned so that these data can be linked as needed with one another and with an individual's medical data. Responsibility for these activities currently falls across research, operational, and personnel organizations and preventive medicine and nuclear, biological, and chemical organizations. DoD should clarify these responsibilities to permit the most effective integration and use of environmental exposure information.

Strategy 2 Recommendations

2.1 DoD should assign single responsibility for collecting, managing, and integrating information on non-battle-related hazards.

2.2 DoD should integrate expertise in the nuclear, biological, chemical, and environmental sciences for efficient environmental monitoring of chemical warfare agents and toxic industrial chemicals for both short- and long-term risks.

2.3 For major deployments and deployments in which there is an anticipated threat of chemical exposures, during deployments DoD should collect biological samples such as blood and urine from a sample of deployed forces. Samples can be stored until needed to test for validated biomarkers for possible deployment exposures or analyzed in near real time as needed for high-risk groups.

2.4 DoD should clearly define the individuals permitted access to and the uses of biological samples and the information derived from them. DoD should communicate these policies to the service members and establish a process to review ethical issues related to operational data collection and use.

2.5 DoD should ensure that adequate preventive medicine assets including laboratory capability are available to analyze deployment exposure data in near real time and respond appropriately.

2.6 DoD should ensure that the deployed medical contingent from command surgeons to unit medics has mission-essential information on the likely non-battle-related hazards of the deployments and access to timely updates.

2.7 DoD should implement a joint system for recording, archiving, and retrieving information on the locations of service member units during operations.

2.8 Environmental monitoring, biomarker, and troop location and activity databases should all be designed to permit linkages with one another and with individual medical records. It is crucial that means be developed to link environmental data to individual records.

STRATEGY 3

Develop the risk assessment, risk management, and risk communication skills of military leaders at all levels.

Military leaders are crucial to the successful preparation and execution of any military mission. Successful leaders are masters of military science, which at its core entails the assessment, management, and communication of battle risk. Although military leaders are well schooled in military science developed for the traditional battlefield, they should be better equipped to address the full range of risks to the health of deployed forces in today's missions. The failure to adequately prepare the leadership for this new milieu may result in reduced mission-readiness and force effectiveness and at times unnecessary exposures to avoidable risks (see Box 2-1). Thus, the training of the leadership in the assessment, management, and communication of health and other non-battle-related

> **BOX 2-1**
> **Exposures to Avoidable Risks**
>
> • Service member concerns about personal protective measures for insects and application of the insect repellent DEET (N,N-diethyl-meta-toluamide) to their skin contributed to several cases of malaria following a deployment to Somalia in 1993 (Newton et al., 1994; Ledbetter, 1995).
> • Also in Somalia, problems arose when family members of injured soldiers learned about firefights and injuries from the news media instead of from more reliable sources of information through the chain of command. Distraught family members in the United States called their relatives who were deployed service members, upsetting the service members and causing decreases in force effectiveness. Commanders developed a system of phone trees to notify family members in near-real time of the status of their family members after a conflict event (LaBoa, 2000).

risks is a mission-essential task. The committee believes that such training will, in time, redress the credibility problems that result as the military attempts to move through this unfamiliar territory on a case-by-case basis.

All levels, but particularly commanders and medical personnel, need training in how health risk assessments are generated and how risk is communicated and managed, taking into account evolving societal concerns. The current guidance provided to commanders and military medical personnel is inadequate because it can result in incomplete and inaccurate descriptions of risk, and thus mismanagement of the risk and insufficient communication about the risk of concern. It does not reflect the most contemporary scientific principles of risk assessment, risk management, and risk communication (Fischhoff, 1995; Leiss, 1996; NRC, 1996).

In recent years, all three services have developed doctrine for operational risk management. The Army's Field Manual FM 100-14, the Navy's OPNAVINST 3500.39 (MCO 3500.27), and the Air Force's Instruction 91-213 and Pamphlet 91-215 all reflect similar approaches to risk assessment. The approach follows the classic risk assessment paradigm established by the NRC "Red Book" in 1983 (NRC, 1983). The book describes a risk assessment process in which the assessment and characterization of a risk are separated from broader social concerns, and the level of participation of the affected communities is low at the initial stages of risk estimation. More recent perspectives have evolved from this traditional paradigm.

In practice, health risk assessment cannot be easily separated from risk management (including risk communication) (NRC, 1996). Moreover, the circumstances and perspectives of those likely to experience the consequences of decisions to be made must influence the process of risk characterization. Characterizations of risk should include consideration of fairness, the context and necessity of exposures, and other factors crucial to human perceptions of risk (NRC, 1996).

To be effective leaders today, commanders must understand these contemporary principles of risk assessment and risk management. They also need to be able to communicate effectively about these topics with the service members they lead and with their families. For example, a traditional model of risk assessment may lead military medical personnel to emphasize the low probability of a negative reaction to a vaccine when attempting to persuade service members to comply with orders to be inoculated. These arguments, however, can actually exacerbate concern if communications leave unanswered the questions most important to individuals. Service members may question the certainty of risk estimates, the effectiveness of inoculation under different deployment scenarios, or the acceptability of any level of risk when the rationale for a vaccine has not been effectively communicated. Furthermore, questions may arise about the fairness of a policy that is perceived to have ignored fears about the long-term consequences of a vaccine.

Effective risk communication is not a simple algorithm, nor is it conducive to checklists.[10] It sometimes requires dialogue instead of the "top-down" information flow common in military settings. Commanders will need to be trained in discussing and hearing the concerns of the individuals in their units about potential health risks. They will also need to turn to their medical staffs and unit medics for additional information about the concerns of their units. This training in risk communication is not a one-shot event but must be ongoing, with continuing reevaluation and effort. DoD trainers in risk communication should continue to draw upon outside experts to ensure the currency of their materials and approaches. Training should be supplemented or updated if a need arises over time or if circumstances change and the risk communication process targets new questions or audiences. Commanders and other risk communicators within DoD should see health risk assessment, risk communication, and risk management as interrelated components of a decision-making process.

The most effective risk communication process must include evaluation of its effectiveness. Box 2-2 provides some considerations that may be useful in evaluating the effectiveness of risk communication.

All of these criteria will not (and cannot) be satisfied in some cases. For example, in the theater of operations, time constraints regarding decision making may exist, making it unproductive, unwise, or undesirable to engage in an extended and explicit consideration of the uncertainties of the risk estimates associated with impending activities. Acceptance, however, of the unavoidable uncertainties of risk management in particular deployment circumstances is more likely with a high level of trust and a belief that troop protection receives top priority. Service members must feel confident that commanders and the military establish-

---

[10]Further discussion of risk communication in the military is found in *Strategies to Protect the Health of Deployed U.S. Forces: Medical Surveillance, Record Keeping, and Risk Reduction* (IOM, 1999, pp. 92–98).

> **BOX 2-2**
> **Considerations Useful in Evaluating**
> **Risk Communication Effectiveness**
>
> An evaluation of the effectiveness of a risk communication process might include the following considerations:
>
> - Are the prioritized concerns of service members and their families reflected in the decision making process and the products of risk assessments?
> - Does risk communication promote and foster trust among service members and their families?
> - Do service members and their families believe that their perspectives have been considered in decision making?
> - Have parties addressed concerns about fairness and equity in the distribution of risk across service members and their families?
> - Have communicators engaged in an open and inclusive process of risk communication?
> - Are service members and their families satisfied that uncertainties associated with scientific estimates of risk have been identified and given serious consideration in the decision making process?
> - Have communications effectively presented the rationale for choices and made clear what dimensions were weighed in formulating decisions related to risks?
> - Has the risk communication process improved the effectiveness of the mission?

ment, as a rule, incorporate service members' perspectives and concerns into risk assessments and decisions. Risk communication training should include some education about the varied contexts in which communication occurs and training in how to identify when a more involved, deliberative process is required.

Physicians and other health care providers also need training in health risk communication so that they can better listen and respond to concerns raised by service members. For many health-related topics, it is helpful for the health care provider to acknowledge both the incompleteness of medical and scientific understanding and the areas where evidence is more complete. **The acknowledgment of uncertainty does not erode trust and confidence in leaders; instead, it fosters confidence in the reliability of information deemed to be more certain and valid.** In addition to training in risk communication for commanders and health care providers, DoD itself must demonstrate greater openness. It should develop an overall plan for risk communication generally that involves stakeholders (the service members and their families) and outside experts and that includes a response plan for new risks to or health concerns of deployed forces (IOM, 1999). This requires an inclusive, iterative process in which assessments and communication approaches are reevaluated in response to input from affected and interested parties (NRC, 1996).

This dynamic approach to risk communication emphasizes ongoing participatory strategies. It suggests that DoD must provide more information to service members and their families than it has in the past, including some of the complexities of risk–benefit trade-offs. It must also immediately admit to mistakes and fully air all the facts related to mistakes as quickly and as transparently as possible. **DoD must be candid with and trusted by service members, their families, and the American people.**

Strategy 3 Recommendations

3.1 DoD should provide training in the contemporary principles of health risk assessment and health risk management to leaders at all levels to convey understanding of the capabilities and uncertainties in these processes.

3.2 DoD should institutionalize training in risk communication for commanders and health care providers. Periodic formal evaluation and monitoring of the quality of training programs should be standard procedure. Risk communication should be framed as a dynamic process that is responsive to input from several sources, changing concerns of affected populations, modifications in scientific risk evidence, and newly identified needs for communication.

3.3 DoD should jump start training in risk communication by delivering it at appropriate settings for various levels of service, including at the time of initial entry into service and at the service schools. DoD should give particular attention to the training of medical officers on initial entry into service. Opportunities for supplemental training and support of ongoing education in risk communication should be formally identified.

3.4 DoD should include the stakeholders (service members, their families, and community representatives) in the development of a plan for DoD risk communication to include when and how risk communications should take place when new concerns arise.

STRATEGY 4

Accelerate implementation of a health surveillance system that spans the service life cycle and that continues after separation from service.

An earlier report (IOM, 1999) dealt at some length with many of the different factors and needs for improvement in the military's health surveillance system. Here, the committee highlights some of the most urgent needs: health history and health status information on recruits, periodic updates of health status information that continue to be obtained after deployments, improved laboratory-based surveillance, and clarified leadership for preventive medicine and health surveillance.

Baseline health information on service members that begins upon their entrance in the military and that is periodically updated is crucial. The Recruit Assessment Program (RAP) (IOM, 1999) is a promising program now in the pilot phase to gather demographic, medical, psychological, occupational, and risk factor data on recruits soon after they begin training. Periodic standardized updates to the medical record[11] are also needed to maintain current and accurate data about service members' health status. The data from all the various health assessments and physical examinations administered throughout the service career must be collected and stored such that they are available to health care providers and epidemiologists as needed, and the survey instruments must be periodically evaluated to ensure that reliable and relevant data are collected. To the extent possible, consistent health domains or dimensions should be measured over the life of the service member.

Reports of health problems in veterans after their deployment to the Gulf War made clear another challenge for military health surveillance: the need to continue to collect health information after the service member has returned from a deployment. An annual health status questionnaire should continue to be administered to those who remain in the military. In the years after a major deployment, the same questionnaire should also be given to a representative sample of those who separate from the military for a period of 2 to 5 years after the deployment. Data collected from those who use health care for the 2 years after a major deployment as part of the Veterans Benefits Improvement Act of 1998 should be captured and used to provide information on the symptoms experienced by this population and the diagnoses made. Extensive and effective cooperation is required between DoD and the U.S. Department of Veterans Affairs (VA) to permit long-term surveillance of the health of deployed forces.[12] The Military and Veterans Health Coordinating Board could facilitate this cooperation.

A crucial aspect to medical surveillance is the timely central reporting of laboratory results. The information systems in current use are insufficient to this task; in particular, the International Classification of Diseases, version 9 (ICD-9)-based reporting is inadequate for infectious disease surveillance (IOM, 1999). Central reporting of laboratory findings as well as provider reporting of clinical

---

[11] Such as through the Health Evaluation and Assessment Review discussed previously (IOM, 1999, pp. 47–48).

[12] The Millenium Cohort Study, now in the planning phase, could help to provide insights on service member health status after deployments.

diagnoses should be required for reportable conditions. It is imperative that DoD be able to provide reliable automated laboratory-based surveillance, with capabilities both to discern and to investigate disease outbreaks. Thus, integration of laboratory and epidemiological expertise is needed.

Many of the topics addressed in this report concern actions and operations that are the responsibility of the preventive and occupational medicine components of the services. For the recommendations in this strategy to be effectively implemented, it is crucial that their efforts be adequately supported with personnel and resources. More physicians are needed who are trained and experienced in preventive medicine (Lane, 2000). Expansion of preventive medicine residencies or other programs such as M.D.-Ph.D. programs is needed to provide the personnel base for military needs. Furthermore, improved coordination of many of their efforts is needed. For example, environmental, infectious disease, psychological-behavioral, and injury-safety considerations all have a bearing on preventive medicine during a deployment and members of these disciplines should not carry out their efforts in isolation. Similarly, laboratory analysis, training, and epidemiological investigations need to be integrated for an effective preventive medicine effort. Strong leadership is needed to better clarify and support the role of preventive medicine within and across the individual services and DoD. Without it, competing systems and a lack of coordinated planning are likely to continue to hamper effective surveillance of the health of the forces and the provision of effective medical support for commanders and the mission.

Strategy 4 Recommendations

4.1 DoD should establish clear leadership authority and accountability to coordinate preventive medicine—including environmental and health surveillance, training, and investigation—within and across the individual services and DoD. DoD should ensure that adequate preventive medicine personnel and resources are available early on deployments.

4.2 DoD should collect health status and risk factor data on recruits as they enter the military, as planned through the Recruit Assessment Program, now in the pilot stage. DoD should maintain health status data for both active-duty and reserve service members with annual health surveys.

4.3 DoD should continue to collect self-reported health information from service members after their deployments to permit comparisons with their predeployment health and with the health of other service members. For a representative sample of those who leave the military health system, DoD should continue to administer the annual health status survey for 2 to 5 years after a major deployment to learn about health changes after deployments.

4.4 DoD should mandate central reporting of notifiable conditions including laboratory findings across the services. DoD should strengthen public health laboratory capabilities and integrate laboratory and epidemiological resources to facilitate appropriate analysis and investigation.

STRATEGY 5

Implement strategies to address medically unexplained symptoms in populations that have been deployed.

Medically unexplained symptoms are symptoms not explained by a known medical etiology that lead to use of the health care system (e.g., chronic fatigue syndrome). The report *Strategies to Protect the Health of Deployed U.S. Forces: Medical Surveillance, Record Keeping, and Risk Reduction* describes how such symptoms are increasingly recognized as prevalent and persistent problems in civilian populations, in which they are associated with high levels of subjective distress and functional impairment with extensive use of health care services (IOM, 1999). Similar conditions have been observed in military populations after military conflicts dating back to the Civil War, and in the absence of increased understanding such conditions are anticipated after future deployments (Hyams et al., 1996; Presidential Advisory Committee on Gulf War Veterans' Illnesses, 1996). The medically unexplained symptoms reported by veterans of the Gulf War have been the driving force behind many expert studies as well as several new programs and initiatives in DoD and VA.

The committee believes that, in addition to the improvements in health surveillance and preventive measures described earlier, DoD's approach to medically unexplained symptoms is another means to address an issue of importance to service members, their families, and the public. It is therefore important that several steps be taken or continued in this area.

First, the ability of military health care providers to identify, communicate with, and manage patients with medically unexplained symptoms must be improved. Although a specific program of primary prevention is not feasible given the current state of knowledge, enough is known to implement a secondary prevention strategy. For example, there is increasing evidence of the effectiveness of cognitive behavioral therapy (CBT) for addressing such symptoms (Buckelew, 1989; Martin et al., 1989; Peck et al., 1989; Salkovskis, 1989; Blanchard et al., 1990; Hellman et al., 1990; Skinner et al., 1990; DeGuire et al., 1992; Keefe et al., 1992; Sharpe et al., 1992, 1996; Payne and Blanchard, 1995; Sharpe, 1995; Speckens et al., 1995; Van Dulmen et al., 1996; Deale et al., 1997; Fulcher and White, 1997; Clark et al., 1998). Studies also indicate that medically unexplained symptoms are more difficult to treat once they have become chronic (Kellner, 1986, 1991; Kroenke and Mangelsdorff, 1989; Craig et al., 1993; Barsky, 1998), providing an additional incentive to identify and treat sufferers early.

Work is under way within DoD to develop a set of clinical practice guidelines for postdeployment health care, including guidelines for the management of chronic fatigue syndrome, which shares many characteristics with other types of medically unexplained symptoms. Once developed, the guidelines will need to be implemented along with research to evaluate their effects on patient outcomes.

DoD has an important opportunity to build on this information base with additional research. Not only can the military health care system explore the effectiveness of management and treatment options by evaluating health outcomes,[13] but it can also expand understanding of some of the predisposing, precipitating, and perpetuating factors for medically unexplained symptoms. This will require the collection of information relevant to medically unexplained symptoms in both the RAP currently being piloted and a periodic health status questionnaire such as the Health Evaluation Assessment Review (HEAR) (IOM, 1999). Beyond simply collecting the information, a research plan for medically unexplained symptoms must be designed and implemented. Since there is no evidence to suggest that medically unexplained symptoms differ between civilian and military populations, research into this topic should be of general benefit. This research should be done with the involvement of both DoD and VA to gain insights into both short- and long-term outcomes. As hypotheses about treatment options and predisposing, precipitating, and perpetuating factors are tested and refined, the information can be used to better protect and promote the health of service members and can be helpful for the general population. If properly designed, the large prospective study of deployed forces (Millenium Cohort Study) now in the planning phases might provide insights into these and other illnesses that may be associated with deployment. Plans should be made for the RAP, HEAR, and Millenium Cohort Study to evaluate similar multidimensional factors relevant to health so that these factors can be assessed over the lifetime of the service member.

New treatment or management guidelines will need to be accompanied by training of the military health care providers. The best setting for the identification and management or treatment of patients with medically unexplained symptoms is in the primary health care setting. Thus, a program of continuing education about medically unexplained symptoms should be undertaken for military primary care providers, as should a program that educates those starting their military medical service in the military graduate medical education programs and the service schools. Care providers must learn to establish working relationships with patients with medically unexplained symptoms so that they understand the current limits of medical knowledge and do not feel dismissed or stigmatized by the lack of an identified medical etiology. At the same time,

---

[13]VA and DoD have under way a large clinical trial that is assessing the benefit of multimodal therapy including CBT and aerobic exercise on the physical functioning of veterans with Gulf War illnesses (VA and DoD, 1999). Completion of the trial is planned for late 2001.

health care providers and the entire system must remain open to new data that might provide insights into medical etiologies for these patients.

Education and discussions about medically unexplained symptoms should not be confined to medical professionals. Misconceptions and ignorance about medically unexplained symptoms exist throughout society, and the military is a microcosm of that society. DoD must squarely face the problem of medically unexplained symptoms. Efforts at the communication of risk to the wider military should include the provision of information about medically unexplained symptoms to remove some of the mystery and fear surrounding them. Like the rest of the general public, service members from commanders on down need to be aware that medically unexplained symptoms are not uncommon in the general population, that they may be more prevalent in service members after military deployments, and that treatments that can prevent or mitigate disability from them are available.

Strategy 5 Recommendations

5.1 DoD should include information about medically unexplained symptoms in the training and risk communication information for service members at all levels.

5.2 DoD should complete and implement guidelines for the management of patients with medically unexplained symptoms in the military health system. DoD should provide primary health care and other health care providers with training about medically unexplained symptoms and in the use of the guidelines. DoD should carry out clinical trials to accompany the implementation of the guidelines and evaluate their impact.

5.3 DoD should establish a treatment outcomes and health services research program within DoD to further provide an empirical basis for improvement of treatment programs to address medically unexplained symptoms. This program should be carried out in collaboration and cooperation with the U.S. Department of Veterans Affairs health system and the U.S. Department of Health and Human Services.

5.4 DoD should design and implement a research plan to better understand predisposing, precipitating, and perpetuating factors for medically unexplained symptoms in military populations.

STRATEGY 6

Implement a joint computerized patient record and other automated record keeping that meets the information needs of those involved with individual care and military public health.

In the 10 years since the Gulf War, insufficient improvements to military medical record-keeping systems have been made. Medical records for service members are contained in a mixture of distinct automated and paper-based systems (National Science and Technology Council, 1998) at multiple and remote locations. There is still no consistent means for documenting in individual medical records ambulatory care that service members receive during deployments (Office of the Special Assistant for Gulf War Illnesses, 1999; COL Mark Rubertone, Director, Army Medical Surveillance Activity, personal communication, March 10, 2000). Progress has been unacceptably slow toward development of the computer-based patient record (CPR) (IOM, 1999) and automated reporting of laboratory results.

A well-functioning medical information system is crucial for the military and crucial for successfully implementing many of the recommendations in this report. Outside experts as well as those within DoD have described the need for an automated system that would fulfill the varied needs of the large DoD health care system (IOM, 1996a, 1999; National Science and Technology Council, 1998; Staggers and Leaderman, 2000), but progress toward the goals has been slow (IOM, 1999).[14] A major challenge is the existence of many separate information systems developed independently to address different needs over the years. Often each branch of the military has its own processes and programs for data collection. The net effect is one of disjointed systems (that often cannot be linked) that are difficult to access and that do not yet successfully fulfill the needs for the entire force. Fewer systems that simultaneously address multiple functions are required. To accomplish this will require strong centralized leadership, careful planning, and coordination.

The committee believes that the design and implementation of a cross-service CPR and related automated systems to support patient care and public health needs are among the most important challenges to protecting the health of deployed forces today. The system must fulfill many needs for many people. The data collected must comply with preestablished standards so that they can be integrated as needed from different systems. A single authority with accountability is mandatory to make this possible in an organization with a strong tendency to create distinct and specialized applications.

---

[14] The Institute of Medicine report by principal investigators Philip Russell and Samuel Guze, *Strategies to Protect the Health of Deployed U.S. Forces: Medical Surveillance, Record Keeping, and Risk Reduction* (IOM, 1999), treats the topic of the military health information systems in more detail and serves as the starting point for this section.

The committee has a particular interest in the medical record systems under development for use during deployments. Some improvements have occurred in this area since the Gulf War, but significant challenges remain, including the use of different systems by different services and the lack of means for the recording of ambulatory medical events in an individual's medical record. Although simple solutions for the most basic medical surveillance needs might be possible fairly quickly, progress on the whole effort is slowed by trying to build a system that can accommodate both current and anticipated future information needs—from simple text to multimedia data and from simple querying facilities to expert systems and decision support systems. The committee urges accelerated implementation of a system for mission critical needs that is consistent with the architecture and data standards planned for the final system instead of waiting for a system that provides total capabilities. The mission critical needs must be defined by preventive medicine and casualty care experts within the military.

Finally, plans for how information on personnel locations, environmental exposure databases, and other databases will be able to interface with the CPR are not yet in evidence. These are crucial aspects of the development of the comprehensive, life-long medical record described as a goal for protection of the health of deployed forces (National Science and Technology Council, 1998). Work is progressing slowly on a means to share medical record information between DoD and VA so that medical records for service members are available to VA health care providers for patients who have separated from the military.

As limited as the progress in medical record keeping has been for the active duty forces, less progress has taken place for reserve forces (Reserve and National Guard). Medical record keeping for reserve forces is the same as that for active-duty forces when they are on deployments, but the real challenge is in maintaining medical information for the reserve forces after or between deployments. Since they receive their medical care from civilian systems, the military has no accessible health status or medical data on these individuals before deployments, beyond the predeployment questionnaire.[15] As a result, individuals among reservist units may needlessly be receiving an additional immunization when reserve units are sometimes immunized en masse (LaBoa, 2000; Lynch, 2000). At a minimum, records of the immunizations provided to service members including members of the reserves need to be stored in individual medical records. Automation of immunization records for all service members should be a priority for the development of the CPR.

---

[15] A more complete description of some of the particular challenges for health surveillance and medical record keeping for reserve forces is found in IOM, 1999, pp. 141–145.

Strategy 6 Recommendations

6.1 DoD should treat the development of a lifetime computer-based patient record for service members as a major acquisition, with commensurate high-level responsibility, accountability, and coordination. Clear goals, strategies, implementation plans, milestones, and costs must be defined and approved with input from the end users.

6.2 DoD should accelerate development and implementation of automated systems to gather mission-critical data elements. DoD should deploy a system that fills the basic needs of the military mission first but is consistent with the architecture and data standards planned for the overall system.

6.3 DoD should implement the electronic data system to allow the transfer of data between DoD and the U.S. Department of Veterans Affairs.

6.4 DoD should establish an external advisory board that reports to the Secretary of Defense to provide ongoing review and advice regarding the military health information system's strategy and implementation.

6.5 DoD should include immunization data, ambulatory care data, and data from deployment exposures with immediate medical implications in the individual medical records and should develop a mechanism for linking individual records to other databases with information about deployment exposures.

6.6 DoD should develop methods to gather and analyze retrievable, electronically stored health data on reservists. At a minimum, DoD should establish records of military immunizations for all reservists. DoD should work toward a computerized patient record that contains information from the Recruit Assessment Program and periodic health assessments and develop such records first for those most likely to deploy early.

References

Army News Service. 1999. Recruiting Ends Year on Positive Trend. *ArmyLink News*, October 5, 1999.

Barsky, A. J. 1998. A Comprehensive Approach to the Chronically Somatizing Patient [editorial]. *Journal of Psychosomatic Research* 45(4):301–6.

Blanchard, E. B., K. A. Appelbaum, C. L. Radnitz, et al. 1990. Placebo-Controlled Evaluation of Abbreviated Progressive Muscle Relaxation and of Relaxation Combined with Cognitive Therapy in the Treatment of Tension Headache. *Journal of Consulting and Clinical Psychology* 58(2):210–5.

Buckelew, S. P. 1989. Fibromyalgia: A Rehabilitation Approach. A Review. *American Journal of Physical Medicine and Rehabilitation* 68(1):37–42.

Clark, D. M., P. M. Salkovskis, A. Hackman, et al. 1998. Two Psychological Treatments for Hypochrondriasis. A Randomised Controlled Trial. *British Journal of Psychiatry* 173:218–25.

Craig, T. K., A. P. Boardman, K. Mills, O. Daly-Jones, and H. Drake. 1993. The South London Somatisation Study I: Longitudinal Course and the Influence of Early Life Experiences. *British Journal of Psychiatry* 163:579–88.

Deale, A., T. Chalder, I. Marks, and S. Wessely. 1997. Cognitive Behavior Therapy for Chronic Fatigue Syndrome: A Randomized Controlled Trial. *American Journal of Psychiatry* 154(3):408–14.

DeGuire, S., R. Gevirtz, Y. Kawahara, and W. Maguire. 1992. Hyperventilation Syndrome and the Assessment of Treatment for Functional Cardiac Symptoms. *American Journal of Cardiology* 70(6):673–7.

DoD (U.S. Department of Defense). 1994. Report of the Defense Science Board Task Force on Persian Gulf War Health Effects. Defense Science Board, Office of the Under Secretary of Defense for Acquisition and Technology, Washington, DC.

DoD. 1997. Implementation and Application of Joint Medical Surveillance for Deployments. DoD Instruction Number 6490.3, August 7, 1997, U.S. Department of Defense, Washington, DC.

Fischhoff, B. 1995. Risk Perception and Communication Unplugged: Twenty Years of Progress. *Risk Analysis* 15(2):137–45.

Fischhoff, B., A. Bostrom, and M. J. Quadrel. 1993. Risk Perception and Communication. *Annual Review of Public Health* 14:183–203.

Fisher, A. 1991. Risk Communication Challenges. *Risk Analysis* 22(2):173–9.

Fulcher, K. Y., and P. D. White. 1997. Randomised Controlled Trial of Graded Exercise in Patients with the Chronic Fatigue Syndrome. *British Medical Journal* 314(7095): 1647–52.

GEO-CENTERS, Inc. and Life Systems, Inc. for the U.S. Army Center for Environmental Health Research. 1997. *Deployment Toxicology Research and Development Master Plan*. U.S. Army Medical Research and Materiel Command, Ft. Detrick, MD.

Hellman, C .J., M. Budd, J. Borysenko, D. C. McClelland, and H. Benson. 1990. A Study of the Effectiveness of Two Group Behavioral Medicine Interventions for Patients with Psychosomatic Complaints. *Behavioral Medicine* 16(4):165–73.

Hyams, K. C., F. S. Wigmall, and R. Roswell. 1996. War Syndromes and Their Evaluation: From the U.S. Civil War to the Persian Gulf War. *Annals of Internal Medicine* 125(5):398–405.

IOM (Institute of Medicine). 1996a. *Health Consequences of Service During the Persian Gulf War: Recommendations for Research and Information Systems*. National Academy Press, Washington, DC.

IOM. 1996b. *Evaluation of the Department of Defense Persian Gulf War Comprehensive Clinical Evaluation Program*. National Academy Press, Washington, DC.

IOM. 1997. *Adequacy of the Comprehensive Clincial Evaluation Program: A Focused Assessment*. National Academy Press, Washington, DC.

IOM. 1999. *Strategies to Protect the Health of Deployed U.S. Forces: Medical Surveillance, Record Keeping, and Risk Reduction*. National Academy Press, Washington, DC.

International Life Sciences Institute. 1993. *Regulating Risk: The Science and Politics of Risk: A Conference Summary*. International Life Sciences Institute, Washington, DC.

The Joint Staff, Medical Readiness Division. 2000. Force Health Protection: Healthy and Fit Force, Casualty Prevention, Casualty Care and Management. The Joint Staff, Medical Readiness Division, Washington, DC.

Kasperson, R. E., and J. X. Kasperson. 1996. The Social Amplification and Attenuation of Risk. *Annals of the American Academy of Political and Social Science* 545:95–107.

Keefe, F. J., J. Dunsmore, and R. Burnett. 1992. Behavioral and Cognitive-Behavioral Approaches to Chronic Pain: Recent Advances and Future Directions. *Journal of Consulting and Clinical Psychology* 60(4):528–36.

Kellner, R. 1986. *Somatization and Hypochondriasis*. Praeger, New York.

Kellner, R. 1991. *Psychosomatic Syndromes and Somatic Symptoms*. American Psychiatric Press, Washington, DC.

Kroenke, K., and A. D. Mangelsdorff. 1989. Common Symptoms in Ambulatory Care: Incidence, Evaluation, Therapy, and Outcome. *American Journal of Medicine* 86(3): 262–6.

Kuehn, R. R. 1996. The Environmental Justice Implications of Quantitative Risk Assessment. *University of Illinois Law Review* 13:103–72.

Kunreuther, H., and P. Slovic. 1996. Science, Values, and Risk. *Annals of the American Academy of Social and Political Science* 545:116–25.

REFERENCES

LaBoa, G. 2000. Report to Committee on Strategies to Protect the Health of Deployed U.S. Forces, Meeting 3, May 24, 2000. Institute of Medicine, Washington, DC.

Lane, D. S. 2000. A Threat to the Public Health Workforce: Evidence from Trends in Preventive Medicine Certification and Training. *American Journal of Preventive Medicine* 18(1):87–96.

Ledbetter, D. 1995. Malaria in Somalia: Lessons in Prevention. *JAMA* 273(10):774–775.

Leiss, W. 1996. Three Phases in the Evolution of Risk Communication Practice. *Annals of the American Academy of Political and Social Science* 545:85–94.

Lynch, BGen. R. 2000. Approaches to Operational Commander Buy-In on Strategies to Protect Forces. Presentation to Committee on Strategies to Protect the Health of Deployed U.S. Forces, Meeting 2, February 8, 2000. Institute of Medicine, Washington, DC.

Martin, P. R., P. R. Nathan, D. Milech, and M. van Keppel. 1989. Cognitive Therapy vs. Self-Management Training in the Treatment of Chronic Headaches. *British Journal of Clinical Psychology* 28 (Pt. 4):347–61.

National Center for Environmental Health. 2000. Preparing for Chemical Attacks by Terrorists. NCEH Pub. No. 99-0499-D [www document]. URL http://www.cdc.gov/nceh/dls/one_pagers/bioterrorism.htm (accessed June 22, 2000).

National Institutes of Health Technology Assessment Workshop Panel. 1994. The Persian Gulf Experience and Health. *JAMA* 272(5):391–6.

National Science and Technology Council. 1998. *A National Obligation: Planning for Health Preparedness for the Readjustment of the Military, Veterans, and Their Families After Future Deployments*. Executive Office of the President, Washington, DC.

Newton J. A. Jr., G. A. Schnepf, M. R. Wallace, L. O. Lobel, C. A. Kennedy, and E. C. Oldfield 3rd. 1994. Malaria in U.S. Marines Returning from Somalia. *JAMA* 272(5):397–399.

NRC (National Research Council). 1983. *Risk Assessment in the Federal Government: Managing the Process*. National Academy Press, Washington, DC.

NRC. 1996. *Understanding Risk: Informing Decisions in a Democratic Society*. National Academy Press, Washington, DC.

NRC. 2000a. *Strategies to Protect the Health of Deployed U.S. Forces: Analytical Framework for Assessing Risks*. National Academy Press, Washington, DC.

NRC. 2000b. *Strategies to Protect the Health of Deployed U.S. Forces: Assessing Health Risks to Deployed U.S. Forces. Workshop Proceedings*. National Academy Press, Washington, DC.

NRC. 2000c. *Strategies to Protect the Health of Deployed U.S. Forces: Detecting, Characterizing, and Documenting Exposures*. National Academy Press, Washington, DC.

NRC. 2000d. *Strategies to Protect the Health of Deployed U.S. Forces: Force Protection and Decontamination*. National Academy Press, Washington, DC.

Office of the Special Assistant to the Deputy Secretary for Gulf War Illnesses. 1999. Information Paper: Military Medical Recordkeeping During and After the Gulf War [www document]. URL http://gulflink:osd.mil/mrk (accessed August 13, 1999).

Payne, A., and E. B. Blanchard. 1995. A Controlled Comparison of Cognitive Therapy and Self-Help Support Groups in the Treatment of Irritable Bowel Syndrome. *Journal of Consulting and Clinical Psychology* 63(5):779–86.

Peck, J. R., T. W. Smith, J. R. Ward, and R. Milano. 1989. Disability and Depression in Rheumatoid Arthritis. A Multi-Trait, Multi-Method Investigation. *Arthritis and Rheumatism* 32(9):1100–6.

Presidental Advisory Committee on Gulf War Veterans' Illnesses. 1996. *Final Report.* U.S. Government Printing Office, Washington, DC.

Reuter, R. 1999. Areas of Additional Potential Consideration in Year 3 Related to the Analytical Framework for Assessing Risk. Presentation to Committee on Strategies to Protect the Health of Deployed U.S. Forces, Meeting 1, November 30, 1999. Institute of Medicine, Washington, DC.

Salkovskis, P. M. 1989. Somatic Problems. Pp. 235–76 in *Cognitive-Behavioral Approaches to Adult Psychiatric Disorders: A Practical Guide.* K. Hawton., P. M. Salkovskis, J. W. Kirk, and D. Clark (eds.). Oxford University Press, Oxford, United Kingdom.

Sharpe, M. 1995. Cognitive Behavioral Therapies in the Treatment of Functional Somatic Symptoms. Pp. 122–43 in *Treatment of Functional Somatic Symptoms*, R. Mayou, C. Bass, and M. Sharpe (eds.). Oxford University Press, Oxford, United Kingdom.

Sharpe, M., R. Peveler, and R. Mayou. 1992. The Psychological Treatment of Patients with Functional Somatic Symptoms: A Practical Guide. *Journal of Psychosomatic Research* 36(6):515–29.

Sharpe, M., K. Hawton, S. Simkin, et al. 1996. Cognitive Behavior Therapy for the Chronic Fatigue Syndrome: A Randomized Controlled Trial. *British Medical Journal* 312(7022):22–6.

Skinner, J. B., A. Erskine, S. Pearce, I. Rubenstein, M. Taylor, and C. Foster. 1990. The Evaluation of a Cognitive Behavioral Treatment Programme in Outpatients with Chronic Pain. *Journal of Psychosomatic Research* 34(1):13–9.

Slovic, P. 1987. Perception of Risk. *Science* 19(5):359–73.

Speckens, A. E., A. M. van Hemert, P. Spinhoven, K. E. Hawton, J. H. Bolk, and H. G. Rooijmans. 1995. Cognitive Behavorial Therapy for Medically Unexplained Physical Symptoms: A Randomised Controlled Trial. *British Medical Journal* 311(7016): 1328–32.

Staggers, N., and A. V. Leaderman. 2000. The Vision for the Department of Defense's Computer-Based Patient Record. *Military Medicine* 165(3):180–5.

VA (U.S. Department of Veterans Affairs) and DoD. 1999. New Research to Help Care for Gulf War Veterans. Brochure. VA Office of Research and Development, August, 1999.

Van Dulmen, A. M., J. F. Fennis, and G. Bleijenberg. 1996. Cognitive-Behavioral Group Therapy for Irritable Bowel Syndrome: Effects and Long-Term Follow-Up. *Psychosomatic Medicine* 58(5):508–14.

APPENDIX A

Study Scope and Statement of Task

STUDY SCOPE

The health of military personnel who served in the Persian Gulf War (PGW), and of those who will serve in future deployments, is a matter of great concern to the veterans, public, Congress, and Department of Defense (DoD). The DoD has requested the advice of the NAS and IOM on a long-term strategy for protecting the health of our nation's military personnel when deployed to unfamiliar environments. The project will draw on the lessons of the Persian Gulf War and subsequent deployments as well as a variety of other evidence to offer recommendations for: (1) an analytical framework for assessing the risks to deployed forces from a variety of medical, environmental, and battle-related hazards, including chemical and biological agents (CBA); (2) improved technology and methods for detection and tracking of exposures to these risks; (3) improved technology and methods for physical protection and decontamination, particularly of CBA; and (4) improved medical protection, health consequences management and treatment, and medical record keeping.

CHARGE TO THE THIRD-YEAR COMMITTEE

In the study's third year, a newly formed committee will use the reports developed by the four respective sets of principal investigators and advisory panels as a starting point to synthesize a final report. In it, the committee will emphasize and extend those findings and recommendations from the interim reports considered to be most important to a long-term strategy for health protection, as well as expanding its review to broader, cross-cutting issues. The committee could examine policy, technology, and organizational issues as necessary in considering a strategy for the future.

Areas of potential emphasis and extension from the interim reports include (but are not limited to):

- Use of a systematic approach to evaluate non-battle risks associated with the activities and settings of deployments;
- Training regarding risk assessment, risk management (including exposure minimization), and risk communication before, during, and after operations;
- Collection and management of environmental data and person location, biological samples, and activity data to facilitate analysis of deployment exposures and to support clinical care;
- Computerized patient records and other automated record keeping that supports patient care and military public health needs;
- Medical surveillance spanning the service life cycle and beyond;
- Strategies to address medically unexplained physical symptoms in deployed populations; and
- The role of military preventive medicine in deployment health.

APPENDIX B

Strategies to Protect the Health of Deployed U.S. Forces: Analytical Framework for Assessing Risks—Executive Summary

Deployment of forces in hostile or unfamiliar environments is inherently risky. The changing missions and increasing use of U.S. forces around the globe in operations other than battle call for greater attention to threats of non-battle-related health problems—including infections, pathogen- and vector-borne diseases, exposure to toxicants, and psychological and physical stress—all of which must be avoided or treated differently from battle casualties. The likelihood of exposure to chemical and biological weapons adds to the array of tactical threats against which protection is required. The health consequences of physical and psychological stress, by themselves or through interaction with other threats, are also increasingly recognized. In addition, the military's responsibility in examining potential health and safety risks to its troops is increasing, and the spectrum of health concerns is broadening, from acute illness and injury due to pathogens and accidents to possible influences of low-level chemical exposures, which can manifest themselves in reproductive health and chronic illnesses years later, perhaps even after cessation of military service.

Some well-publicized cases have led to scrutiny of the military's procedures for identifying potential hazards and for collecting the information on hazards, exposure, and health-status surveillance that is necessary to detect and monitor threats to the troops' health and welfare.

To help prevent and reduce the number of illnesses in future deployments, the Department of Defense (DoD) asked the National Academy of Sciences (NAS) to advise it on a long-term strategy for protecting the health of the nation's military personnel when deployed to unfamiliar environments. In response to this request, a collaborative effort was established between the Institute of Medicine (IOM) and the National Research Council (NRC) and four tasks were identified as key to addressing DoD's request. They were: (1) develop an analytical framework for assessing health risks to deployed forces; (2) review and evaluate technology and methods for detection and tracking of exposures to potentially harmful chemical and biological agents; (3) review and evaluate technology and methods for physical protection and decontamination, particularly of chemical and biological agents; and (4) review and evaluate medical protection, health consequences management and treatment, and medical record keeping.

This report addresses the first task of developing an analytical framework for assessing risks, which would encompass the risks of adverse health effects from battle injuries, including those from chemical- and biological-warfare agents, and the non-battle-related health problems noted above. The presumed spectrum of deployment ranged from peacekeeping to full-scale conflict.

APPROACH TO THE CHARGE

This report was prepared by Dr. Lorenz Rhomberg of Gradient Corporation (formerly of the Harvard School of Public Health), with the help and guidance of 10 advisers who represented various scientific disciplines, including military operations, toxicology, infectious diseases, use of biomarkers, personal exposure assessment, epidemiology, occupational health, psychiatry, and risk assessment (see Appendix B). The group received briefings, reviewed documentation of current DoD practices, considered existing risk-assessment paradigms, and commissioned the preparation of papers on six topics that required in-depth analyses (see Appendix A for abstracts of these papers).

The focus of this report is principally on risk assessment—the identification, characterization, and quantitative description of threats and the impacts they may produce—rather than on the means to control or manage those impacts. It must be borne in mind, however, that such risk assessment must occur within the military context, aimed at enhancing the health and safety of troops while ensuring their military effectiveness, both strategically (through improvement of equipment, doctrine, training, and preparedness) and in actions taken during specific deployments. While the risk assessment framework recommended in this report does not directly address how to put its characterizations of threats to use in risk-management decision-making, it does attempt to steer the conduct of risk-assessment activities so as to provide the most useful and appropriate information while avoiding critical gaps.

Because of the diversity of threats that the recommended framework must be able to address, it cannot be very specific about any one activity, and it does not try to be a flowchart or decision tree that maps out a process, step by step. The term "framework" as used herein means an organized context for conducting assessment activities that defines the relationship of the component activities to the achievement of the larger aims of protecting the health of deployed forces. Rather than a prescription of a specific program or a plan for its implementation, the framework is a set of strategies for conducting risk-assessment activities so as to be most useful to the military's needs. Accordingly, emphasis is placed on examining how those needs differ from the more widely familiar context of environmental risk assessment. The NRC's 1983 risk-assessment paradigm forms the core of the framework, providing a structure for analysis and characterization of particular exposures to particular hazards. The framework recommended herein expands the scope of the paradigm, by showing that the structure can address not only toxic chemicals, but also such other threats as risks of microbial infections, mechanical failures, transportation accidents, and tactical threats. The particular technical methods will vary with the nature of the threat under analysis, and the framework includes ways of modifying standard approaches to be applicable to military situations.

The framework must go beyond the NRC paradigm to organize the process of recognizing how the varied activities entailed in deployment of forces might lead to exposures to hazards that need analysis, cataloging these, setting priorities among them for analysis, analyzing them, and integrating the results so as to yield a comprehensive risk-management program that addresses the full array of threats with which troops must deal during deployment.

Threats to deployed forces can be assessed with the tools developed in the civilian risk-assessment context, but it must be recognized that the military context differs. Many hazards are specific to military situations, military exposure factors can differ from those relevant to civilians, and stress and extreme environments can affect toxic responses. A useful management scheme must address all the threats that deployed troops face, so integration is particularly needed. The military mission has primacy, and its needs might dictate that troops bear risks that would not be acceptable in a civilian setting. Extraordinary measures to protect against threats to health and safety can encumber military effectiveness or increase vulnerability, so well-thought-out tradeoffs among military and nonmilitary concerns are necessary. Risk information must be presented in a way that permits rapid decisions to be made in the field by commanders with little pertinent technical expertise.

For many hazards relevant to military deployments, the concern is not for continuous low-level exposures, but for episodes that occur as a consequence of unplanned and unpredictable events, such as equipment failures, actions by an adversary, and collateral damage of chemical-storage facilities. Risk analysis for such hazards must focus as much on describing the likelihood of toxicologically important exposures as on the responses to exposures. One can analyze such exposures by tracing scenarios leading to exposure of troops and by examining the likelihood that key precipitating events occur, whether they be physical occurrences or actions on the part of adversaries or of the deployed forces themselves. The problem can often be divided into the likelihood that a potential hazard is in the deployment area, the likelihood of release of a hazard into the environment, the likelihood of exposure of troops to the released material (based on fate and transport modeling), and the likelihood of adverse health effects, given the exposure (based on dose-response analysis).

No attempt is made in this report to assess particular individual risks or to critique the current DoD systems or established risk-assessment practices, nor is any attempt made to create a comprehensive catalog of threats. The risks of injury from conventional weapons or nuclear weapons are not addressed herein, and psychological stress is addressed only in general, because of the lack of established ways to assess the risk of such stress. This omission is a shortcoming of the risk-assessment framework recommended in this report, since psychological stress is a factor of major importance to the health of deployed forces and deployment veterans, and any solution to how DoD should approach disorders and unexplained symptoms among veterans must include consideration of the contribution of stress. Further work on this topic is recommended.

A risk-assessment framework should be a means to help achieve DoD's program objectives for addressing the health and safety risks to deployed forces, so such objectives must be clearly defined. It is provisionally suggested that they should include minimizing the impact of disease and non-battle-related injuries; developing a straightforward and systematic program to address risks and executing the program efficiently; diligently and competently addressing health and safety threats; integrating risk awareness and the appropriate weighing of risks and benefits into decision-making; improving the ability to characterize risks posed by past exposures; and doing all the foregoing in the light of cost and effects on military capability and effectiveness. The recommended framework attempts to bring the methodology of risk assessment to bear on these objectives.

The process should be open, encouraging scrutiny of DoD actions and the incorporation of health and safety concerns into all aspects of decision-making. Emphasis should be placed on proactive recognition of potential threats, and characterizing and setting priorities for them; monitoring for detection and characterization of known threats and their impacts; and ongoing and retrospective surveillance of troops' (and veterans') health status for effects that may arise despite protective efforts.

DESCRIPTION OF THE FRAMEWORK

The recommended framework is a structured approach to gathering, organizing, and analyzing information in a way that encourages a comprehensive, integrative assessment and response to the threats that deployed troops might face. Unlike more traditional risk assessments, the recommended framework is concerned with examining *activities* (such as deployment near an industrial facility that stores various toxic chemicals) rather than *specific threats*. Focusing on the threats associated with particular military deployment activities, rather than specific threats, encourages thinking beyond a standard list of recognized hazards, facilitates redesign of practices and materiel to mitigate risks, and avoids increasing one risk to reduce another. By emphasizing planning and attention to previously uncharacterized threats, the framework aims to minimize the likelihood of overlooking important risk factors. Characterizing the effects of various levels of exposure, as opposed to simply defining "safe" levels, increases the ability to make appropriate tradeoffs.

The recommended framework for risk assessment of threats to deployed U.S. forces is composed of three phases, which are characterized by the timeline of deployment: ongoing, deployment, and post-deployment (see Table B-1).

Ongoing Strategic Preparation

The ongoing strategic baseline preparation phase of the framework involves all the activities and analyses undertaken to prepare for threats in future deployments. The activities are not tied to particular deployments, but represent the need for continuing development of information about potential deployment risks and exposures, organized through the framework so as to create an ever expanding and improving base of knowledge. This knowledge can be drawn upon to increase the capability to avoid or mitigate risk and to refine doctrine and training so as to lead to safer deployments.

TABLE B-1 Framework for Phases of Risk Assessment

Ongoing Strategic Baseline Preparation
   Anticipation of potential threats and circumstances
   Priority-setting for detailed analyses
   Risk analysis
   Incorporation of results into planning

During Deployment
   Deployment-specific planning
   Initial activities
   Continued deployment
   Activities to terminate deployment

Post-Deployment
   Reintegration of troops
   Data archiving
   Continuing health surveillance
   Population analyses of exposure effects
   Evaluation of lessons learned

Ongoing preparation has four steps: anticipating potential threats and the circumstances under which they might arise, setting priorities among the potential threats for analysis, conducting qualitative and quantitative risk analyses of the threats, and incorporating the resulting risk estimates into exposure guidelines and planning. In the first step, established lists of hazardous threats (such as toxic chemicals, infectious disease agents, insecticides, and vaccines) are reviewed, and threats with notable exposure patterns are examined. Potential threats can be identified by constructing deployment scenarios and placing hazards in three categories: those associated with deployment-specific activities (such as heat stress), those associated with particular types of missions (such as peacekeeping and ground combat), and those associated with particular locations (such as climate, indigenous diseases, and local pollution). In addition to identifying potential exposures to threats, the scenario-drawing process helps to link exposures directly to the activities that cause them and to delineate chains of events that lead to particular outcomes. It is important to consider in this step the potential for coexposures (such as vaccinations, antidotes, and pesticides) that could lead to accumulative or synergistic effects.

Once the potential threats to deployed troops are identified, priorities must be set for analysis. That is done by examining the most likely deployment scenarios and determining which hazards are most likely, which are mission-critical (would affect the chance of success of the military mission), which constitute known threats, which could have widespread or severe effects, and which are peculiar to the deployment setting—all features that suggest priority attention.

Once the hazards and the circumstances under which they might arise are identified and ranked, the traditional tools of risk assessment can be used to develop quantitative or qualitative risk estimates. In the dose-response analysis, consideration should be given to potential interactions with other threats, the duration of exposure, and the importance of dose-rate effects. For each potential hazard, it is also important to examine the possible scenarios that lead to an adverse outcome and to recognize that some scenarios require a chain of events to produce the outcome, in which case the probability of each scenario is based on the probabilities of the separate events.

An important step in the ongoing strategic baseline preparation phase of the framework is the incorporation of the risk-assessment results into planning, design of doctrine and standard operating procedures, and training. For example, exposure standards can be established for achieving some degree of protection under different circumstances (such as short-term emergency exposures and chronic low-level exposures). Because detailed risk analysis can be time-consuming, appropriate generic analyses and contingency plans that can quickly be adapted to and implemented in actual deployment situations should be formulated. Such formulations should take account of the fact that different deployment missions will have different spectra of tactical risk, as well as different opportunities and costs for health protective measures.

During Deployment

The second major phase of the framework addresses risk-assessment activities associated with actual specific deployments, either as case-specific pre-deployment planning preparation or as activities conducted during the course of deployment. The key activities associated with this phase are implementing plans made in anticipation of deployment (ongoing strategic baseline preparation and planning), refining them with information peculiar to the specific deployment, noting the advent of threatening exposures, and activating the appropriate parts of the response plans accordingly. This phase must also include vigilance for exposures that, despite all the planning, were unanticipated. DoD should examine the effectiveness of collecting and archiving biological samples, in addition to sera, from troops and environmental samples for future analysis. Such information could provide rapid results during deployment so that risk management can be continually refined. This information could also validate and refine baseline strategies.

When a specific deployment is expected, information on its location, mission, and current conditions should be incorporated into predesigned generalized contingency plans. This includes information on meteorological conditions and forecasts, updates on the locations of hazardous materials, and current assessments of capabilities and inclinations of adversaries. A plan to obtain information on potential exposures during the course of deployment should be specified; its extent will depend on the nature, magnitude, and anticipated duration of the specific deployment. On arrival at a deployment destination, samples of soil, air, and water should be obtained and tested for local pollutants, and some samples should be archived for future reference. In addition, detection devices for the most likely threats and meteorological instruments should be set up to obtain information for use in exposure models.

Over the course of the deployment, various kinds of information should be collected periodically (with the extent of the activity depending on the deployment specifics): environmental samples to document changes in environmental concentrations, information on unit activities and positions, and information collected by monitors and detectors. DoD should examine the effectiveness and feasibility of collecting biological samples during deployment. It is also important during the course of deployment to be vigilant for novel and unanticipated threats.

The information collected during deployment is valuable for retrospective analyses, such as reconstruction of exposure scenarios, comparisons with pre-deployment health surveys and samples, and improvement in contingency plans. These data constitute an important source of information for investigating health issues that might arise among deployment veterans.

After Deployment

Post-deployment risk assessment is the third major phase of the framework. In this phase, the health of deployment veterans is monitored for later-appearing effects, and analyses are conducted to ascertain whether these effects are associated with exposures experienced during deployment.

DoD should consider the effectiveness of collecting and archiving health information and biological samples after deployment for the purpose of follow-up and retrospective analyses to address questions about illnesses that might arise later. Surveillance of veterans' health should be continued, and uncertain outcomes should be investigated with exposure reconstruction and epidemiologic analyses. Much of the information obtained about threats during this phase of the framework can be used to refine the ongoing strategic baseline risk analyses by providing a deeper understanding of known threats and by identifying threats not previously considered.

RECOMMENDATIONS

The risk-assessment framework presented in this report should be used by DoD as a basis for organizing its efforts and learning what kinds of work are needed for the protection of the safety and health of forces deployed in hostile environments.

What will make the framework most useful is not the execution of each of its elements, however competently done, but rather the systematic approach to the process of assessing threats to deployed troops and incorporating the results of each element of analysis into an integrated program that addresses the overall objectives of the troop health protection program.

In implementing the framework, DoD should

- Develop an explicit list of objectives, such as those described in this report, for efforts to protect the health and safety of deployed forces and to periodically assess progress in meeting the objectives.
- Strive to examine and reexamine as warranted all the effects of a given hazardous agent or threat, not only the effects that were first known, including risks posed by low exposures that could eventually lead to chronic illness.
- Continue to conduct research on methods to address different magnitudes, durations, patterns, and coexposures that might be encountered during deployment.
- Develop risk-assessment methods to characterize and predict effects of psychological and physical stress in potentiating or exacerbating the physical, chemical, and biological effects of hazardous agents or threats and as hazards in their own right.

APPENDIX B 53

- Conduct research and develop methods to assess risks posed by exposure to microbial agents, and strive to characterize the variety of disease organisms that might be encountered around the world and troops' vulnerability to them.
- Examine patterns of coexposure to various threats; because deployment is characterized by many simultaneous exposures, develop methods to assess possible effects of combinations of threats and their interactions with stress; and develop methods to identify the combinations that should receive further scrutiny based upon biological considerations, because they are peculiar to specific kinds of deployment, or because of particular DoD responsibilities.
- Make special efforts to identify previously unrecognized hazards by examining deployment activities and settings for potential threats and by identifying scenarios that might lead to hazardous exposures.
- As an aid to decision-making in emergencies related to particular hazardous substances, compile and make readily accessible the exposure levels and durations at which people are expected to begin to suffer progressively severe effects.
- Conduct expert analyses before deployment to update general scenarios with case-specific details for quick application by field commanders.
- Conduct research on developing appropriate biological markers of exposure and effect for surveillance of exposures that are of particular relevance to the deployment setting.
- As part of the tracking of troops' exposures and activities, DoD should consider the effectiveness of collecting and archiving biological samples, in addition to sera, from troops and environmental samples before, during (if warranted and feasible), and after deployment.
- Conduct annual health evaluations of reserve and active-duty personnel to obtain baseline health information, as recommended in the companion IOM report addressing medical surveillance.
- Develop an explicit framework for risk-management decision-making that would use information obtained from the application of the risk-assessment framework.

APPENDIX C

Strategies to Protect the Health of Deployed U.S. Forces: Detecting, Characterizing, and Documenting Exposures— Executive Summary

BACKGROUND

Since Operation Desert Shield/Desert Storm, Gulf War veterans have expressed concerns about the health effects associated with possible hazardous exposures during their service. In response, several expert bodies have conducted extensive studies and recommended improvements in U.S. Department of Defense (DoD) policies, procedures, and technologies for protecting military personnel during deployments. Recently, the National Academies was also asked to conduct an independent, external, unbiased evaluation of DoD's efforts to protect deployed forces and to provide advice on a long-term strategy for protecting the health of deployed U.S. military personnel.

The complete evaluation involves four areas: risk assessments; technologies for detecting and tracking exposures (the present study); physical protection and decontamination; and medical surveillance, record keeping, and risk reduction. These four preliminary studies will provide a basis for a synthesis report by a subsequent National Academies committee.

Task of This Study

The objectives of this study are listed below:

- Assess current and potential future approaches used by DoD for detecting and tracking exposures of military personnel to potentially harmful agents, including chemical and/or biological (CB)[1] warfare agents and other harmful agents.

• Evaluate the efficacy and implementation of current policies, doctrine, and training and identify opportunities for adjusting or augmenting strategies to provide better protection in future deployments.

• Review and evaluate tools and methods for tracking and characterizing inventories of CB agents in the deployed theater; for tracking and characterizing the locations and time-activity patterns of deployed military personnel; for detecting and monitoring concentrations of potentially harmful agents; for estimating exposure concentrations and patterns of exposure for individuals or groups; and for implementation (e.g., documenting exposures).[2]

Conduct of the Study

The principal investigator, an expert in exposure assessment, conducted the study with the help of National Research Council (NRC) staff, who collected data, and an advisory panel that reviewed the report while it was being developed and furnished additional information. Other sources of information included reports and databases of regulatory and research organizations, experts in relevant disciplines, meetings with DoD representatives, and reviews of relevant documents (e.g., field manuals) and literature.

Study Approach

This study focuses on technologies for detecting and monitoring concentrations of agents and for tracking exposures of troops to those agents. The study also includes a review of the overall framework in which these technologies could be used. No attempt was made to assess the budgetary impact on DoD of adopting some or all of the recommendations in this report. The study excludes the many computing, information processing, data storage, and communications technologies being developed, mostly in the private sector. DoD's use of these technologies has been investigated in many other reports; and it is widely agreed that future military systems for command, control, communications, intelligence, surveillance, and reconnaissance will require new technologies to meet the growing demand for sensor integration, high-speed data transport, additional

---

[1] In this report, the acronym CB refers to chemical and/or biological agents that can be used as weapons.

[2] In this study, the terms detecting, monitoring, and tracking are differentiated as follows. Detecting is the process of determining the presence of agents. Monitoring is the process of collecting data to develop space and time profiles of agent concentrations. Tracking provides information on both the geographic locations of troops and on their activities at those locations (e.g., marching, operating inside a vehicle, sleeping in a tent, or eating).

data storage, and data distribution and analysis to achieve full, real-time, situational awareness on the battlefield and meaningful postdeployment assessments. If the recommendations in this study are implemented, they could add significantly to DoD's existing needs for improving computers, information processing and storage, and communications technologies.

This report is intended to assist DoD in coping with issues raised by exposures before, during, and after future deployments. Because data documenting past experiences are limited and variable, this report recommends a prospective strategy for handling exposure-related issues in future deployments.

Military Doctrine and Training

For many years the military has adhered to a doctrine of contamination avoidance, which involves four steps: (1) implementing passive defensive measures (e.g., camouflage, dispersion) to reduce the probability of exposures to CB agents; (2) warning and reporting attacks with CB agents to protect others who might be affected; (3) locating, identifying, tracking, and predicting CB hazards to enable commanders to decide whether to operate in spite of them or to avoid them; and (4) limiting exposures of personnel if operation in a contaminated area is deemed necessary. According to military guidance documents, avoiding CB hazards completely is the best course of action; but this is not always possible. Thus, military personnel are trained in the use of protective gear (e.g., masks and suits). Although operating effectively in a CB environment is extremely difficult, the military believes that well trained troops can survive and fight on a contaminated battlefield.

Although the military offers substantial guidance for protecting personnel against chemical attacks, it also acknowledges that its detection capabilities (especially for biological agents) are limited and is working to improve its equipment. As recently as 1996, troops were told to treat any future suspected biological attack like a chemical attack and to rely on protective masks, although then-current detector systems would not react to biological agents. Although contamination avoidance is still the guiding principle of CB doctrine, the military is also developing concepts for CB defense. The focus of CB defense will certainly change as technologies and threats evolve and as troops are deployed to areas where toxic industrial hazards are known to be present. Training goals for the future include virtual, live, and simulated training exercises, modeling and simulations (e.g., of agent dispersion), and specialized training in protecting troops against military and industrial toxic agents.

CHARACTERIZING EXPOSURES

Characterizing the effects of exposures to harmful agents is vital for defining the level of protection necessary for operations in contaminated areas and for providing postexposure medical treatment. Characterizing exposures requires detecting the presence of agents, assessing and monitoring agent concentrations, tracking time-specific locations of troops relative to these concentrations, and determining exposure pathways. Although all of these information sets are treated in this report, no single information set can provide sufficient information for characterizing exposures in real time or for completely characterizing potential or past exposures. As discussed below, information sets must be combined to be useful for decision makers.

Monitoring agent concentrations requires a system that can detect and record both concentrations and environmental factors, such as wind, that can affect the spread and concentration of agents. Perhaps the best way to monitor the movement of an agent is with a combination of a monitoring network and dispersion simulations. However, even detailed information on space and time distributions of concentrations is not sufficient to characterize troop exposures; the location of the troops in relation to the concentration, the rate and direction of their movements, and their degree of protection must also be known. Ideally, every individual should be tracked in real time, but this may not be practical in the near future. Modeling and war games can be used to help determine the feasibility of eventually tracking every individual. For now and in the near future, however, units could be tracked by tracking a representative sample of individuals in that unit.

DoD is aware that it must be able to anticipate significant exposures to CB agents and other harmful agents in future deployments. Therefore, DoD is currently devoting significant resources to improving its capabilities of anticipating health-threatening exposures. DoD is also aware of the need to collect and store information on low-level exposures to CB agents and other harmful substances. The low-level issue involves not only improved technology and equipment, but also interpreting trends from measurements collected near the detection limits of equipment and using exposure data for a representative fraction of the exposed population.[3]

Finding: To date, exposure assessments for both civilian and military populations have focused primarily on exposures to contaminants in a specific medium (e.g., air, water, soil, food) or on exposures to specific environmental pollutants. DoD's current plans for monitoring CB agents would also be limited to a specific medium and would not be time-space specific, would not include time-activity records, and would not account for both short-term and long-term expo-

---

[3]If tracking and exposure information on individuals could be temporarily stored and retrieved at a later date for historical purposes, this would alleviate the near-term problems of data overload and provide an option for determining later the effects on individuals of low-level exposures to CB agents. A high-capacity version of the Personal Information Carrier now under development by the Army might provide these capabilities.

sures. These factors would only be included in settings where deployed personnel were active (in garrisons or in the field).

Most of the sampling protocols included in CB agent reconnaissance operations are designed to provide comprehensive area coverage, rather than statistical sampling or stratification. DoD has not systematically evaluated how modeling, simulations, and decision analysis could be used in real time to anticipate acute exposures (especially imminent threats). DoD's current capabilities and strategies have not been structured for making optimum use of these tools.

Recommendation: The Department of Defense (DoD) should devote more resources to designing and employing both statistical sampling and sample stratification methods. Two useful examples of probability-based statistical sampling are the National Human Exposure Assessment Studies (NHEXAS) and Total Exposure Assessment Methodology (TEAM) studies. DoD should modify these sampling techniques to meet its needs and should evaluate how modeling, simulations, and decision analysis could be used in real time to anticipate acute exposures.

Finding: Personal passive monitoring of atomic radiation, in the form of dosimeters and radiation badges, has been successfully used for many decades. In some limited situations, small passive monitors have also been used to detect chemicals. However, current technology limits personal monitoring of many toxic gases and particulate matter to the use of active monitoring, which is a complex process.

Recommendation: The Department of Defense should explore and evaluate the use of personal monitors for detecting chemical and biological agents, toxic industrial chemicals, and other harmful agents at low levels. If all personnel were equipped with monitors, probabilistic sampling could be used to select a subset of data for short-term, immediate use (e.g., to define the contaminated parts of the deployment area). The full data set could be used for long-term purposes (e.g., recording an individual's exposure to low-level toxic agents). Stratification of the subsets should be decided on the basis of exposure attributes, such as location, unit assignment, and work assignment. If the logistics problems can be solved, every deployed person could ultimately wear a personal monitor.

Finding: DoD is currently devoting significant resources to improving its capabilities of monitoring life-threatening exposures but not of significant exposures to other harmful agents. At this time, DoD also recognizes the value of, but has taken little action, to collect and store information on low-level exposures to CB agents, toxic industrial chemicals (TICs), environmental and occupational contaminants, and endemic biological organisms. Different capabilities will be required for detecting life-threatening exposures, monitoring low-level exposures to CB and industrial agents, monitoring potential exposures to harmful microorganisms, and maintaining complete exposure records for all military personnel.

Recommendation: The Department of Defense (DOD) should rank the threat levels of all known harmful agents and exposure pathways based on the dimensions of harm (e.g., health consequences, the number of personnel affected, the time to consequences). When assessing the need for and applications of new equipment, increased surveillance, and improved documentation, DoD should include these data, and, if applicable, use decision analysis methods, such as probabilistic decision trees, to make decisions and prepare operations orders.

THRESHOLDS OF HEALTH EFFECTS

Measures of safe and unsafe doses have been established for high-level exposures to both CB agents and TICs. Information on dose responses for low dose rates and long-term exposures to chemical agents is still sparse. In addition, exposures to biological agents have been much more difficult to detect and measure than exposures to chemical agents. For chemical agents, a low-level exposure is one that does not result in acute effects. However, over the long term, low-level exposure may increase the likelihood of chronic illness. In contrast to high-level exposures, for which clear evidence of health effects exists, as low-level chemical exposures increase, it is postulated that the probability of disease increases. Risks from chemical agents have been assessed, but risks from biological agents have not. Therefore, it is difficult to define a low-level exposure to biological agents. Although an acute threshold concentration for chemical agents can be characterized and a safety factor establishing a low-level exposure can be applied, this information is rarely available for biological agents.

Finding: Because little information is currently available to relate long-term health effects to low-dose or low-dose-rate exposures to chemical agents, it is extremely difficult to set performance criteria for detecting and monitoring concentrations of these agents to assess long-term health effects. As a starting point for a working definition of low-level concentration, DoD could use the low-dose data currently available and the capability of available detection equipment.

Recommendation: The Department of Defense (DoD) should increase its efforts to collect and evaluate individual and group dose-response data for a broad set of chemical warfare agents. Studies could include standard animal toxicity testing protocols for long-term effects, as well as retrospective epidemiological studies on individuals exposed to these substances in their occupations. DoD should use the detection capability of available equipment as its working definition of low-level concentration.

Finding: In addition to chemical warfare agents, thousands of TICs are in or are brought into the theater of deployment. These chemicals include pesticides, fuels, paints, and lubricants. Under combat conditions, existing controls and safety precautions may not be practical. Storage tanks, production facilities, pipelines, and other equipment may be damaged, for example, and the TICs dispersed. Exposure under these conditions may be uncontrolled, unreported, unrecorded, and extremely dangerous. Exposures could have long-term health effects that cannot be easily distinguished from the long-term health effects of low-level exposures to chemical warfare agents.

Detecting and monitoring exposures continually to the full set of toxic chemicals, would be extremely difficult, if not impossible. Toxicity data for a number of TICs being developed by some government agencies, such as the Environmental Protection Agency (EPA) and the Occupational Safety and Health Administration (OSHA), are being reviewed by independent groups, such as the NRC Committee on Toxicology. The data thus far show large variations in toxicity.

Recommendation: The Department of Defense should review its current efforts to catalog and prioritize toxic industrial chemicals. This information should be used to anticipate the types of chemicals that may be encountered during a deployment and to prioritize them.

Finding: Very little information is currently available to relate long-term health effects to low-level exposures to biological agents. Almost no information is available on how combined or sequential exposures to low levels of CB agents can affect the short-term or long-term health of troops. Until DoD can accumulate and analyze information on low-level exposure or dose response, as well as on long-term chronic effects, it will be very difficult to set performance criteria for detecting and monitoring concentrations of CB agents for assessments of long-term health effects. Potential interactions among agents add to the difficulty. Interactions can be cumulative, synergistic, or antagonistic. For example, chemical interactions may, in fact, abate, or even destroy, a biological agent. In fact, at one time, DoD research focused on using a chemical agent to counter a biological agent cloud.

Recommendation: The Department of Defense should increase its efforts to collect and evaluate low-level dose-response data for a broad set of biological agents. The data should include information on the infectivity of a range of both warfare and endemic biological agents. At the same time, studies should be undertaken to determine whether and which combined chemical and/or biological agent exposures should be investigated. This information should be used for defining a strategy for monitoring exposures to multiple agents.

Finding: Current criteria for detecting CB agent concentrations are designed to prevent exposures to lethal and incapacitating levels. Often the only way to determine if individuals have been affected by exposures to harmful agents is if they have immediate symptoms. Thus, data are not provided in a form that can be used to establish or verify retrospectively the health effects of CB agents over the long term.

Recommendation: The Department of Defense should establish a plan to collect data for all types of potential agent exposures to identify potential or emerging medical problems quickly. If possible, these medical problems should then be evaluated in terms of any prior exposures to chemical and/or biological warfare agents that have been associated with that health outcome. This plan should include guidelines for who should get the information and when they should receive it.

ENVIRONMENTAL AND EXPOSURE PATHWAYS

Potential environmental exposure pathways are important considerations of a strategy to protect the health of deployed forces. In an overt attack with CB agents, the inhalation path, and to a lesser extent, the dermal path, are obvious exposure pathways. However, when assessing low-level, long-term, or episodic exposures to either CB agents or TICs, persistent and indirect pathways must also be investigated. Total exposure assessments must take into account ambient concentrations of harmful agents in multiple environmental media (e.g., air, water, solid surfaces), as well as the time and activity patterns and microenvironments of individuals. Exposure can only be quantified when pathways and routes that account for a substantial fraction of the intake have been identified.

Unfortunately, much of the current data on environmental contaminants cannot be synthesized into an understandable form because no comprehensive framework has been developed for evaluating chemical transport, transformation, and interactions in multiple media. Another important aspect of a credible exposure assessment is the possibility of concurrent or sequential exposures. Tracking these exposures can be a complex undertaking, especially if the agents interact synergistically or antagonistically.

Finding: During deployment, troops may be exposed to multiple harmful agents from multiple sources at various concentrations. Therefore, measurements and models must be designed to evaluate the factors that affect the multipathway intake of pollutants released from single or multiple sources. In preparing a detection and monitoring strategy for the large number of potentially harmful agents and the variety of pathways by which a person can come in contact with agents, priorities must be set on combinations of agents and pathways. Past experience can provide valuable information for ranking threats, but the list should also include plausible threats that have not been encountered in past deployments.

Recommendation: The Department of Defense should develop a portfolio of exposure threats that can be used to set priorities (based on the dimensions of harm), to distinguish between short-term and long-term hazards, and to establish plausibility. Developing this portfolio is likely to require the cooperation of other federal agencies, such as the Food and Drug Administration, the Environmental Protection Agency, the National Oceanographic and Atmospheric Administration, and the Centers for Disease Control and Prevention. The decision-making strategy should include probabilistic techniques to ensure that it is applicable to situations with many uncertainties and rapid changes.

Finding: Combined exposures to drugs, vaccines, chemical substances, and biological substances have been suggested as causal factors for the symptoms among Gulf War veterans. Gulf War veterans had ample opportunities to be exposed to these substances in many different combinations, and interactions can be cumulative, synergistic, or antagonistic.

The risk assessment community has done very little research to provide exposure assessments of the combined health impacts of even two interacting agents.

Recommendation: The Department of Defense (DoD) should begin scientific studies to measure interactions among chemical and/or biological agents and industrial chemicals. DoD's analysis of the effects of mixed-agent exposures should include toxicological studies on mixtures and epidemiological evidence of mixed-agent effects.

DETECTING AND MONITORING HARMFUL AGENT CONCENTRATIONS

CB agents can be detected and monitored in several ways: (1) point and area sampling; (2) local, stand-off, and remote detection; and (3) real-time and delayed analysis. In assessing technologies and detection and monitoring equipment, it is important to consider whether they can provide information on both long-term and short-term (e.g., acute effects that could immediately affect a unit's ability to fight) health effects. Until recently, the focus has been only on short-term affects.

Technologies and equipment are evaluated for accuracy, reliability, sensitivity, selectivity, speed, portability, and cost. Two very different kinds of information are essential during a deployment: (1) real-time detection of harmful agents; and (2) monitoring and archiving of low levels of agent concentrations for postdeployment assessments.

APPENDIX C

Many harmful agents are dispersed as aerosols or attached to aerosols. Detecting them requires either collecting and analyzing the aerosol particles or using particle spectrometry. Currently, mass spectrometry is used to characterize atmospheric aerosols in an attempt to provide on-line, real-time analysis of individual aerosol particles. However, results of current systems are questionable. Current detection methods involve isolating particles on filters and subsequent analysis performed in the laboratory. The isolation processes often disturb the aerosol, which renders the data questionable because the chemicals on particles can evaporate or react before analysis. To overcome these difficulties, technologies such as aerosol time-of-flight mass spectrometry (ATOFMS) have been developed to eliminate the need for filters and chemical collection.

Current mass spectrometers weigh a few hundred pounds and are, therefore, not easily portable. Ion-mobility spectrometers (now under development) may weigh only 10 pounds. Other developments could also improve spectrometers. In addition to basic mass spectrometry, DoD is investigating surface acoustic wave (SAW) and light detection and ranging (lidar) technologies to detect CB agent aerosols. The information provided by this equipment will require data evaluation systems to sort and assess the large amount of information.

Current and planned detection equipment is primarily designed to detect nerve and blister chemical agents. TICs have not been given as high a priority. Most technologies that can detect chemical agents in air, water, and food, however, can be adapted to detect TICs and other harmful chemicals likely to be found in the deployment environment. The SAW detector, for example, would have a limited capability of detecting TICs and other harmful chemicals.

Although the current capability to detect biological agents is limited, developing that capability has recently been given a high priority. Emerging technologies for detecting and identifying microorganisms include polymerase chain-reaction amplification, microchips, molecular beacons, electrochemiluminescence, biosensors, mass spectrometry, and flow cytometry.

Finding: Overall, the technologies and equipment either in use or under development are severely limited in their ability to measure concentrations associated with long-term health risks. A significant reason for this problem is that no formal requirements have been established for detecting and monitoring low-level, long-term exposures. Until acceptable low-dose exposures are specified, performance goals for low-dose detection technology cannot be established. Specifications would provide designers, developers, and operators of detection and monitoring equipment with goals for their research.

Recommendation: The Department of Defense should establish criteria for detecting and monitoring low-level exposures to chemical and biological warfare agents and toxic industrial chemicals. These criteria should specify three detection levels: (1) immediate, dangerous, and life-threatening hazards; (2) short-term hazards; and (3) long-term health risks.

Finding: Because different technologies have different strengths and weaknesses, no single technology should be relied on for detection. By using complementary and redundant technologies and sensor fusion techniques, which are commonly used in other areas of the military (e.g., air defense and antisubmarine warfare), the risk of false alarms could be reduced, and agents could be detected at lower limits.

Recommendation: At least two different but complementary technologies should be used, along with sensor fusion techniques, for the detection of a given type of agent. This combination could significantly reduce the number of false positives and false negatives.

Finding: Most of the equipment currently available, as well as most of the equipment under development, for sensing CB agents is designed for detection and warning only. Detection devices typically give off audible or visible signals when the concentration is above the sensitivity level of the device or above a preset value. These devices are valuable for protecting troops from immediate harm but do not provide the kind of monitoring needed to assess less-than-debilitating exposures or to assess exposures that might lead to delayed health impacts.

Not enough attention has been given to archiving the measurements from different detectors. In some cases, archiving is not possible because of the nature of the device. Devices operated for "warning-only" cannot be used in combination with systems like the multipurpose integrated chemical alarm and Joint Warning and Reporting Network (JWARN) to determine the spatial and temporal trends in agent concentrations—essential information for determining the evolution of a threat or for confirming the absence of an agent.

Recommendation: The Department of Defense should develop a comprehensive plan for collecting and archiving data and samples based on a matrix of short-term threats and long-term health risks for situations before, during, and after deployment. This matrix could be used to prioritize types of information.

TRACKING DEPLOYED MILITARY PERSONNEL

A full characterization of an individual's exposure requires knowing where that person is and what (s)he is doing. General-population, time-activity data cannot be used for estimating exposures of deployed troops; only data specific to deployed personnel can yield accurate estimates of exposures. These data can be provided by the global positioning system (GPS), the total isolated microenvironment exposure (TIME) monitor, and various motion sensors and data loggers, which have been recently introduced.

The GPS will help greatly with the location of units and even of individual soldiers. Miniaturized instruments would have to be developed for use in the field. A wristwatch style GPS, for example, combined with a miniaturized data logger, would provide activity and location information that could be used to prevent acute exposures, as well as to estimate long-term exposure. The most promising automated approach for obtaining data for estimating long-term exposures appears to be a modified TIME device or similar data logger combined with GPS.

Finding: GPS is a critical component of an effective system for predicting and preventing exposures to CB agents, including accidental agent releases. Currently, only one individual per unit or squad carries a GPS receiver. Once GPS devices have been miniaturized and militarized, each individual could carry one. The location of each individual and the individual's proximity to identified or suspected releases of CB agents could then be identified, and orders for preventive actions could be directed to the individuals at greatest risk.

Recommendation: The Department of Defense should continue to support the development of miniature (e.g., wristwatch style) military GPS receivers. Given current technology, receivers could be fielded within five years. The actual decision to equip every deployed unit or individual with a GPS-based receiver should be based on the results of trade-off analyses.

Finding: A miniaturized, multifunctional device that can detect CB agents and TICs, determine location and time, and record the data would be extremely valuable both for protecting deployed troops and for analyzing past exposures. These devices could detect threats from harmful substances, locate the wearer in time and space, and store the data until it could be downloaded. There are, of course, many technical challenges (e.g., size, weight, power requirements) to achieving this capability. Very small devices already exist, however, that could partly meet these goals. The Army's Man-in-Simulant Test (MIST) Program, for example, uses a passive sampler no thicker than a common adhesive bandage and less than one inch square. Establishment of a goal to develop these devices would offer, at a minimum, a valuable target for researchers and developers.

Recommendation: The Department of Defense should support the goal of developing a miniaturized, multifunctional device for detecting agents, determining location, and storing data.

Finding: Individuals may have performed jobs prior to or during their deployment that involved higher-than-average or longer-than-average exposures to toxic pollutants. Predeployment information could be used to identify individuals whose prior exposures put them at higher risk from additional exposures during deployment, as well as to identify possible prior exposures to harmful agents that otherwise might be believed to have occurred during deployment. The postdeployment information would provide a concise record of major duties performed and the use of, or proximity to, possible or confirmed sources of pollutants.

Recommendation: The Department of Defense should implement measures to identify individuals whose predeployment exposures might put them at higher risk of harm from additional exposures during deployment. The information should include major duties performed and the use of, or proximity to, possible or confirmed sources of pollutants during deployment.

STRATEGY

DoD should modify its overall strategy in two ways: (1) by increasing the emphasis on detecting and monitoring concentrations of biological agents during troop deployments; and (2) by addressing the detection and monitoring of a broader range of CB and TIC concentrations and tracking low-level exposures to them in an integrated, systematic way. These two changes will require that DoD take the following steps:

- Develop and procure the technical means of assessing potential and actual exposures (e.g., real-time, field-usable devices for detecting biological agents and improved devices for detecting chemical agents).
- Develop doctrine and training protocols based on improved knowledge of CB exposures for conducting military operations.
- Collect information on the postdeployment health of troops, whether or not they remain in the military.

Defining Needs

Recommendation: The Department of Defense should formulate an integrated approach to assessing the threats of chemical and/or biological agents. The approach should include: (1) a near-term and long-term perspective; (2) data collection; (3) estimates of the relative importance of various threats (e.g., biological threats, chemical threats, and chemical toxins derived from organisms) in a variety of overseas theaters; and (4) data on the effects of low-level doses of a broad range of agents.

Determining Exposure

Recommendation: The Department of Defense (DoD) should proceed with a robust program to develop chemical detectors and biological detectors that can detect and measure low-level as well as high-level concentrations. The first priority should be the development of improved passive sampling devices based on existing technologies that could be fielded quickly. The DoD should also develop a support structure for using the devices and for archiving the data.

Recommendation: The Department of Defense should expeditiously develop the capability of identifying and archiving continuous data on the operational location of each small unit—and, if practical, each individual—as well as the unit or individual's proximity to actual or suspected releases of potentially harmful agents. Technical assessments and cost-benefit analyses should be used to determine the best ways to accomplish these functions in the near term (e.g., the best way of supplementing the miniature global positioning system receiver to achieve the desired result).

Recommendation: The Department of Defense should establish a long-term goal to develop very small devices that could be deployed with each individual to measure and record automatically exposures to one or more of the most threatening agents, the location of the individual, the activity of the individual, the microenvironment, and the time.

Recommendation: The Department of Defense should develop and field improved meteorological measuring and archiving systems to provide finer data grids of wind, temperature, and atmospheric stability in the theater of operations. These data will be necessary for improved transport modeling and for after-action analyses of data on the movements of chemical and biological "clouds."

Recommendation: The Department of Defense should support research to clarify how chemical and biological processes affect the rate of transformation of agents in different environmental media under a variety of conditions.

Handling Data

Recommendation: The Department of Defense should develop a representative activity-location database for different types of units, major military duty categories, and high-risk subpopulations of personnel likely to be deployed. This database, along with models and simulations, should be used to provide insights about potential exposures associated with specific deployments.

Recommendation: The Department of Defense should develop its data-handling capability to track the locations of all individuals (or, at least, the smallest units) during future deployments and compare them to the locations of actual or potential agent concentrations at the same point in time. The data-storage capacity should be increased simultaneously so that these locations can be recalled and analyzed after each deployment (e.g., data could be recalled from a high-capacity personal information carrier).

Recommendation: In the future, the Department of Defense should characterize the variations in exposures of members of groups believed to have been exposed during their deployment. To help accomplish this, location data and agent-concentration data that pertain to individuals or small units should be analyzed thoroughly, using statistical methods where applicable.

Recommendation: The Department of Defense should study the ramifications of establishing a national chemical and biological hazardous agent data center.

Doctrine, Training, and Administration

Recommendation: Doctrine and training for taking protective action should be reviewed to ensure a proper balance between military necessities and the risks of harmful exposures. The Department of Defense should reevaluate its doctrine and training for handling and reporting alarm activations and false alarms and revise them, if necessary.

Recommendation: Doctrine and training should take account of predeployment exposures that might put some individuals at greater risk during deployment. This information, along with data gathered on actual or suspected exposures or on the locations of individuals or units and the locations of concentrations of agents, should be used to assess the risk to individuals.

Recommendation: The Department of Defense should review its doctrine and training protocols governing the interactions of offensive operations and protective measures. If an offensive operation may cause exposure to troops nearby, this information should be factored into the decision.

APPENDIX D
Strategies to Protect the Health of Deployed U.S. Forces: Force Protection and Decontamination— Executive Summary

Since Operation Desert Shield/Desert Storm, Gulf War veterans have expressed concerns that medical symptoms they have experienced could have been caused by exposures to hazardous materials or other deployment-related factors associated with their service during the war. Potential exposure to a broad range of chemical and/or biological (CB) and other harmful agents was not unique to Gulf operations but has been a component of all military operations in this century. Nevertheless, the Gulf War deployment focused national attention on the potential, but uncertain, relationship between the presence of CB agents in theater and health symptoms reported by military personnel. Particular attention has been given to the potential long-term health effects of low-level exposures to CB agents.

Since the Gulf War, U.S. forces have been deployed to Haiti, Somalia, Bosnia, Southwest Asia, and, most recently, Kosovo, where they were (and are) at risk of exposure to toxic CB threats. The U.S. Department of Defense (DoD) anticipates that deployments will continue in the foreseeable future, ranging from peacekeeping missions to full-scale conflicts. Therefore, the health and preparedness of U.S. military forces, including their ability to detect and protect themselves against CB attack, are central elements of overall U.S. military strength. Current doctrine requires that the military be prepared to engage in two simultaneous major regional conflicts while conducting peacekeeping operations and other assignments around the globe. The diversity of potential missions, as well as of potential threats, has contributed to the complexity of developing an effective strategy.

BACKGROUND

In the spring of 1996, Deputy Secretary of Defense John White met with the leadership of the National Academies to discuss the DoD's continuing efforts to improve protection of military personnel from adverse health effects during deployments in hostile environments. Although many lessons learned from previous assessments of Operation Desert Shield/Desert Storm have been reported, prospective analyses are still needed: (1) to identify gaps and shortcomings in policy, doctrine, training, and equipment; and (2) to improve the management of battlefield health risks in future deployments.

DoD determined that independent, external, unbiased evaluations focused on four areas would be most useful: (1) health risks during deployments in hostile environments; (2) technologies and methods for detecting and tracking exposures to harmful agents; (3) physical protection and decontamination; and (4) medical protection, health consequences and treatment, and medical record keeping. This report, which addresses the issues of physical protection and decontamination, is one of four initial reports that will be submitted in response to that request.

CHARGE

This study, conducted by two principal investigators with the support of an advisory panel and National Academies staff from the Commission on Engineering and Technical Systems, assessed DoD approaches and technologies that are, or may be, used for physical protection—both individual and collective—against CB agents and for decontamination. This assessment includes an evaluation of the efficacy and implementation of current policies, doctrine, and training as they relate to protection against and decontamination of CB agents during troop deployments and recommends modifications in strategies to improve protection against deleterious health effects in future deployments. This report includes reviews and evaluations of the following topics:

- current protective equipment and protective measures, as well as those in development;
- current and proposed methods for decontaminating personnel and equipment after exposure to CB agents;
- current policies, doctrine, and training for protecting against and decontaminating personnel and equipment in future deployments;
- the effects of using current protective equipment and procedures on unit effectiveness and other human performance factors; and
- current and projected military capabilities to provide emergency response to terrorist CB incidents.

THREAT AND RISK ASSESSMENT

Chemical and Biological Battle Space

Chemical agents were first used extensively as military weapons during World War I. CB weapons programs continued to flourish during the 1950s and 1960s, led by scientists in the United States and the Soviet Union, and to a lesser extent, in other countries including Great Britain. New nerve agents were developed during those years, including the family of V agents, which are not only lethal in smaller ingested doses but can also be absorbed directly through the skin. Natural toxins and biological pathogens were also investigated as biological warfare agents.

In the post-1950s era, improving the means of dissemination of lethal agents became a major research objective. Airborne spray tanks, specialized artillery shells, CB-capable missile warheads, and an assortment of other weapons were developed. The United States discontinued its offensive biological and chemical military research programs in 1969 and 1989, respectively, but continued to expand its defensive programs. However, CB technologies have continued to proliferate in other countries, and with advances in bioengineering and molecular biological capabilities, even small nations or groups now have the potential to develop novel biological agents. This asymmetrical threat prompted the United States to extend its CB defense programs, which have increased substantially since Desert Shield/Desert Storm.

The estimated CB threat from Soviet forces during the Cold War was based on the perceptions that a broad range of chemical and biological weapons had been fielded, that the Soviet Union had the capability of deploying and supporting those weapons on the battlefield, and that the Soviets were pursuing an extensive research program. U.S. tactics, training, and requirements were based on this perceived threat. Today, many countries possess CB capabilities although intelligence assessments indicate that most of them have limited quantities of agents and limited delivery systems.

Response to Chemical/Biological Threats

The CB threat to U.S. forces can be defined as the perceived capability of an opposing force to expose U.S. forces to CB agents. The most obvious way to minimize the risk of CB exposure is to avoid contact with these materials. Therefore, the military has developed a doctrinal principle for protecting deployed forces based on avoiding exposure (i.e., contamination avoidance). Avoiding contact depends on the capability and availability of detection equipment; however, because of current lag times in detection capability, a responsive strategy (the so-called "detect to treat" strategy), rather than a preventive strategy, has been necessary.

The U.S. intelligence community provides data, analyses, and advice concerning the development of CB capabilities by threat nations. Based on this information, commanders and the Joint Service Integration Group (JSIG) evaluate how CB agents could be used against U.S. troops and develop policy, doctrine, training, and requirements for equipment to counter the perceived threat. As the threat changes, U.S. approaches to countering the threat should also change.

As a result of the proliferation of CB capabilities, recent reductions in U.S. forces, continuing budget constraints, and attempts to minimize duplications of effort among the services, operations have become more integrated and cooperative (i.e., joint service operations). To encourage the integration of CB research and development (R&D) at all levels, in 1994 Congress enacted Public Law 103-160, the National Defense Authorization Act for Fiscal Year 1994 (Title XVII), establishing a new structure for the CB defense program.

Finding: Joint structure and joint service processes were developed to maximize the efficient use of funds and reduce duplications of effort.

Finding: The object of the joint prioritization of system needs (and, therefore, research, development, and acquisition [RDA] needs) is to ensure that fielded systems meet joint service needs. This requires that commander-in-chief (CINC) priorities and nuclear, biological, chemical (NBC) community priorities be coordinated.

Finding: The prioritization and selection of RDA projects are often based on compromises or political trade-offs unrelated to CINC prioritization, technical capabilities, or bona fide needs and are focused on service-specific rather than joint service needs.

Recommendation: The Department of Defense should reevaluate and possibly revise its prioritization process for the development of equipment. The reevaluation should include reassessment of the use of threat information.

Challenge

The chemical agent challenge established for protective equipment ($10 g/m^2$ for liquids; 5,000–10,000 mg-min/m^3 for vapors) has not been changed in four decades. Although analyses using relatively sophisticated computer models have shown that under certain conditions, 10 g/m^2 levels may be present in localized areas of a battlefield, the average concentration may be considerably lower. These same models predict that the areas where levels would be higher than 10 g/m^2 would be the same areas where the shrapnel and projected shell materials would be more likely to cause injuries or deaths than CB agents. Nevertheless, because challenge levels determine the requirements for protection, the goals of the entire CB R&D program are based on the 10 g/m² level for liquid agents and 5,000–10,000 mg-min/m³ for vaporous agents.

Finding: The battlefield areas with the highest contamination levels will also have the highest levels of ballistic fragmentation lethalities. Therefore, CB protective measures will be ineffective in these areas regardless of the liquid or vapor challenge levels. The threat from CB weapons relative to other battlefield threats is unknown.

Finding: System development is sometimes based on outdated and possibly inaccurate evaluations of threats and challenges.

Recommendation: The Department of Defense should reevaluate the liquid and vapor challenge levels based on the most current threat information and use the results in the materiel requirements process and, subsequently, in the development of training programs and doctrine.

Finding: Little or no new funding is being provided for basic research on new technologies for physical protection or decontamination.

Recommendation: The Department of Defense should reprogram funds to alleviate the shortfall in basic research on new technologies for physical protection and decontamination.

PHILOSOPHY, DOCTRINE, AND TRAINING

The CB defense program involves (1) contamination avoidance (reconnaissance, detection, and warning); (2) force protection (individual and collective protection and medical support); and (3) decontamination. Before systems for detecting contaminated areas were available, military planners developed a doctrine (best described as the "fight dirty" doctrine) that was based on conducting operations in contaminated areas. Implementing the doctrine involved providing a combination of individual protective equipment and extensive training on fighting in contaminated environments. As technology has advanced, especially detection technologies, and as new detection equipment has been fielded, the doctrine has shifted to "contamination avoidance." Stated simply, this doctrine provides that U.S. forces will engage an enemy while avoiding casualties from contamination by CB agents.

Once the doctrine of contamination avoidance (with concomitant detection and protective equipment) was adopted, training was naturally modified to carry out the new doctrine. A critical requirement for deterring the use of CB agents (and for successful operations if deterrence fails) is that forces be fully trained to respond to the full spectrum of CB threats. Operational requirements must balance the risk factors from all sources and determine trade-offs between protecting the individual and maintaining the combat effectiveness of the force.

Finding: The current doctrine is based on the concept of contamination avoidance, although U.S. CB detection systems do not, as a rule, provide sufficient advance warning to prevent exposures.

Finding: Unit commanders receive little training related to assessing CB risks to their units, especially in determining when, whether, and how much protective gear is necessary.

Recommendation: The Department of Defense should develop commander training protocols and/or simulations to assist unit leaders in making appropriate chemical and biological risk-based decisions.

INDIVIDUAL PROTECTION

The military conceptual approach to individual protection, called mission-oriented protective posture (MOPP), is an ensemble comprised of protective garments, boots, masks, and gloves. MOPP levels proceed (i.e., adding parts of the ensemble) from the MOPP-ready level to the MOPP 4 level, increasing the level of protection in response to the hazard. Because design requirements for personal protective equipment (PPE) include the ability to withstand the established threat and risk levels, PPE has severely limited individual (and unit) performance. Problems include difficulties in speech and communications, impairment in hearing, reduced vision, thermal stress, occasional adverse reactions to materials, and overall reductions in operational effectiveness.

Some improvements in PPE have been made, however. For example, the joint service lightweight integrated suit technology (JSLIST) affords better CB protection, reduces the physiological heat burden, and interferes less with weapons systems than previous technologies. The JSLIST preplanned product improvement (P3I) should provide even better protection. Because the human respiratory system is extremely vulnerable to the highly toxic and rapidly acting agents to which deployed forces may be exposed, respiratory protection is a major factor in contamination avoidance. Respirators of various types have been developed and used both in military and civilian operations. The newest mask—the joint service general purpose mask (JSGPM)—allows better peripheral vision, is reasonably comfortable to wear, and has a somewhat flexible design to meet service-specific requirements.

The hands have traditionally been protected by impermeable gloves; however, recent research has also focused on multilaminate technologies and barrier creams designed to prevent or reduce the penetration and absorption of hazardous materials by the skin, thus preventing skin lesions and/or other toxic effects.

APPENDIX D 75

Effective barrier creams might also be used to protect skin adjacent to areas where the garments are known to provide less than optimal protection (e.g., under seams, around closures).

Finding: Current challenges used to evaluate protective equipment do not reflect changes in threat levels.

Recommendation: The Department of Defense should reevaluate its requirements for materiel development to protect against liquid and vapor threats and revise design requirements, if appropriate.

Finding: PPE modules (e.g., masks, garments, gloves) were designed as independent items and then "retrofitted" to create an ensemble. They were also developed without adequate attention to various human factors issues, such as the integration of PPE with weapon systems.

Finding: The most serious risk from most CB agents appears to be from inhalation. Current doctrine allows for Mask-Only protection, but the mask seal could be broken while advancing from Mask-Only to MOPP 4 status.

Recommendation: A total systems analysis, including human factors engineering evaluations, should be part of the development process of the personal protective equipment system to ensure that the equipment can be used with weapon systems and other military equipment. These evaluations should include:

- the performance of individuals and units on different tasks in various realistic scenarios, and
- the interface of the mask and garments and potential leakage during an "advance" from Mask-Only to MOPP 4 status.

Finding: Although researchers have good data from human factors testing that identified serious performance (cognitive and physical) limitations as a result of wearing PPE, they have been unable to adequately relate these deficiencies to performance on the battlefield.

Recommendation: The Department of Defense should place greater emphasis on testing in macroenvironments and controlled field tests rather than relying mostly on systems evaluations for personal protective equipment.

Finding: Although the seal of the mask is much improved over previous mask models, seal leakage continues to be a critical problem. The leakage can be attributed to (1) problems with the interface between the seal and the face, and (2) improper fit.

Recommendation: Additional research is needed on mask seals and mask fit. The research program should focus on seals, fit, and sealants (adhesives). The duration/severity of leaks, if any, during transitions in protective posture from one MOPP level to another should also be investigated. These data would be useful for future studies on long-term health effects of low-level exposures. In addition, training to fit masks properly should be conducted for all deployed forces equipped with mission-oriented protective posture equipment.

Finding: Although mask fit testing has been shown to improve protection factors 100-fold, the Air Force and Army have only recently begun deploying mask fit testing equipment and providing appropriate training protocols and supportive doctrine.

Recommendation: Doctrine, training, and equipment for mask fit testing should be incorporated into current joint service operations. The Department of Defense should deploy the M41 Mask Fit Test kit more widely.

Finding: Leakage around closures in personal protective equipment remains a problem.

Recommendation: The Department of Defense should continue to invest in research on new technologies to eliminate problems associated with leakage around closures. This research could include the development of a one-piece garment, the use of barrier creams on skin adjacent to closure areas, and other technologies still in the early stages of development.

Finding: Current gloves reduce tactile sensitivity and impair dexterity.

Recommendation: The Department of Defense should evaluate using a combination of barrier creams and lightweight gloves for protection in a chemical and/or biological environment. Multilaminate gloves should also be further explored.

Finding: An impermeable garment system is believed to provide the most comprehensive protection against CB agents. But impermeable barriers cause serious heat stress because they trap bodily moisture vapor inside the system. Permeable systems, which breathe and allow moisture vapor to escape, cannot fully protect against aerosol and liquid agents.

An incremental improvement could be achieved by using a semipermeable barrier backed with a sorptive layer. This system would allow the moisture vapor from the body to escape and air to penetrate to aid in cooling. The multilayer system would have some disadvantages, however. It would be bulky and heavy. The sorptive layer is an interstitial space where biological agents could continue to grow because human sweat provides nutrients for biological agents, which could prolong the period of active hazards. Countermeasures should be investigated to mitigate these problems.

Recommendation: The Department of Defense should investigate a selectively permeable barrier system that would be multifunctional, consisting of new carbon-free barrier materials, a reactive system, and residual-protection indicators.

The carbon-free barrier materials could consist of: (1) smart gel coatings that would allow moisture/vapor transport and would swell up and close the interstices when in contact with liquid; (2) selectively permeable membranes that would allow moisture/vapor transport even in the presence of agents; (3) electrically polarizable materials whose permeability and repellence could be electronically controlled.

The reactive material could be smart, carbon-free clothing with gated membranes capable of self-decontamination. A reactive coating could also be applied to the skin in the form of a detoxifying agent (e.g., agent reactive dendrimers, enzymes, or catalysts capable of self-regeneration).

A residual-protection indicator would eliminate the premature disposal of serviceable garments and might also be able to identify the type of contamination. Conductive polymers could be used with fiber-optic sensors to construct the device.

COLLECTIVE PROTECTION

Collective protective structures (e.g., shelters and positive pressure vehicles) provide relatively unencumbered safe environments where activities such as eating, recovery, command and control, and medical treatment can take place. Collective protective equipment is based on filtering and overpressurization technologies. Advanced filters and adsorbents are critical components in these systems. Improvements in protection will depend on the availability of advanced filtration and adsorbent capabilities.

Finding: The Department of Defense does not have enough collective protection units to meet the needs of deployed forces.

Recommendation: The Department of Defense should assess the needs of deployed forces for collective protection units in light of changing threats and the development of new personal protective equipment and provide adequate supplies of such equipment to deployed forces.

DECONTAMINATION

Decontamination is the process of neutralizing or removing chemical or biological agents from people, equipment, and the environment. For military purposes, decontamination must restore the combat effectiveness of equipment and personnel as rapidly as possible. Most current decontamination systems are labor intensive and resource intensive, require excessive amounts of water, are corrosive and/or toxic, and are not considered environmentally safe. Current R&D is focused on the development of decontamination systems to overcome these limitations and effectively decontaminate a broad spectrum of CB agents from all surfaces and materials. Because of the vastly different characteristics of personnel, personal equipment, interior equipment, exterior equipment, and large outdoor areas, situation-specific decontamination systems must be developed.

DoD has developed doctrine and training for decontamination but has not established levels of acceptable risk. Therefore, detection capabilities are not designed to verify acceptable decontamination levels.

Finding: Just as only a few benchmarks for the removal of MOPP gear have been established (because detection technology is inadequate), few benchmarks of decontamination levels have been established. Therefore, it is difficult to know when it is safe to return equipment to operational status and impossible to "certify" that previously contaminated equipment can be transported to a new location, especially a location in the United States.

Recommendation: The Department of Defense should initiate a joint service, interagency, and international cooperative effort to establish decontamination standards. Standards should be based on the best science available and may require the development of new models for setting benchmarks, especially for highly toxic or pathogenic agents.

If residual decontamination levels are based on ultraconservative toxicity and morbidity estimates, returning contaminated equipment becomes impractical. Benchmarks for decontamination should be based on highly accurate, reliable, up-to-date toxicity data.

Finding: Although significant progress is being made with limited resources in exploring decontamination technologies that may be effective, no organized, integrated research program has been developed to meet the new challenges and objectives that have been posed (i.e., environmentally acceptable decontamination). Various agencies are actively pursuing many projects, but they are not well coordinated and do not have clear priorities for fixed-site programs, casualty management, and sensitive equipment programs.

Recommendation: The Department of Defense (DoD) should coordinate and prioritize the chemical/biological research and development (R&D) defense program, focusing on the protection of deployed forces and the development of environmentally acceptable decontamination methods. DoD should also establish the relative R&D priority of decontamination in the chemical/biological defense program.

Finding: Recent developments in catalytic/oxidative decontamination (enzymes, gels, foams, and nanoparticles) appear promising for decontaminating a wide range of CB agents.

Recommendation: Research on enzyme systems for battlefield decontamination (especially for small forces) should be given high priority because they could be used to decontaminate both personnel and equipment and would not require large volumes of water or complicated equipment.

Recommendation: The Department of Defense should continue to develop other catalytic/oxidative systems for larger-scale decontamination. If possible, these systems should be less corrosive and more environmentally acceptable than current methods.

Finding: Low-power plasma technology has been shown to be effective for decontaminating sensitive equipment and has the potential of incorporating contaminant-sensing capabilities.

Recommendation: The Department of Defense should continue to develop plasma technology and other radiation methods for decontaminating equipment.

TESTING AND EVALUATION

Testing and evaluation of equipment, methodologies, and the toxicological effects of chemical agents are critical for the development of appropriate defensive strategies. Adherence to the principles of the nonproliferation agreements entered into by the United States prohibits most tests using live agents, as well as studies with human volunteers (except with surrogate agents). Most human and animal tests are, therefore, conducted using simulants, although it is not entirely clear that these simulants are adequate surrogates.

The most comprehensive test program, the Man-in-Simulant Test (MIST) Program, which tests complete and partial protective ensembles under controlled conditions, is a valuable program, although it has many shortcomings. Simulants are commonly used for testing protective and decontaminating equipment to determine the effectiveness of the protective equipment. However, the simulants have not been systematically validated to determine how closely their behavior mimics the behavior of actual agents. Therefore, the United States may not have the ability to determine whether or not a specific piece of equipment actually meets its performance requirements.

Finding: Testing of dermatological threat agents has not been consistent. The available quantitative data are not sufficiently precise to make an accurate evaluation of potential percutaneous threats from agents other than blister agents or irritants.

Recommendation: Tests of dermatological threat agents should be conducted to establish the level of protection necessary to provide adequate margins of safety and to establish quantitative criteria for evaluating the performance of protective equipment, such as gloves, undergarments, and overgarments.

Finding: Mask testing under the MIST program was unreliable because the passive dosimeters did not function satisfactorily in the mask environment.

Recommendation: Active samplers or improved passive samplers for mask testing using simulants should be developed and made available for tests of the joint service lightweight integrated suit technology (JSLIST) ensemble.

ASSESSMENT OF MILITARY CAPABILITIES TO PROVIDE EMERGENCY RESPONSE

Various initiatives have been implemented and numerous studies undertaken to determine the role and assess the capability of the U.S. military in providing emergency response capabilities in coordination with other federal, state, and local agencies. Examples of military programs to support emergency response include the DoD Chemical Biological Rapid Response Team, the U.S. Army Medical Research Institute of Chemical Defense Chemical Casualty Site Team, the Marine Corps Chemical Biological Incident Response Force, and the National Guard Rapid Assessment and Initial Detection Program.

Finding: Because numerous agencies will respond to a domestic CB incident, close coordination will be necessary for the response to be efficient and effective. Unless civilians (e.g., first responders, employees of relevant state and local agencies, etc.) who respond to domestic CB incidents are equipped with protective and decontamination equipment that is compatible with the equipment used by the military, coordination will be difficult if not impossible.

Recommendation: The Department of Defense, in collaboration with civilian agencies, should provide compatible equipment and training to civilians (e.g., first responders, employees of relevant state and local agencies, etc.) who respond to domestic chemical and/or biological incidents to ensure that their activities can be coordinated with the activities of military units. Doctrine and guidance must be developed on an interagency basis.

Finding: Doctrine and training are not well developed for mission-critical civilians working at military installations that might become targets of chemical and/or biological attacks.

Recommendation: Coordinated doctrine, training, and guidance on individual protective equipment, collective protective equipment, and decontamination should be established on a joint service, interagency, and coalition basis for civilians working at military installations.

SUMMARY AND GENERAL RECOMMENDATIONS

The health of military personnel who served in the Gulf War, and of personnel who will serve in future deployments, is a matter of great concern to veterans, the public, Congress, and DoD. Based on the many lessons that have been learned from the Gulf War and subsequent deployments, as well as on information from other sources, a great deal can be done to minimize potential adverse health effects from exposure to CB agents and to increase protection levels against them.

Recommendation: Threat projections and risk perceptions should be reevaluated in terms of realistic or credible battlefield risks. The requirements for protective equipment should then be adjusted to respond to those threats and challenges.

Characterizing a "low-level" contaminated environment is still an open question. Answering this question has become an urgent priority since post-Gulf War medically unexplained symptoms have become a serious issue. Information on the effects of extended exposures to low levels of CB agents is incomplete, but recent studies have suggested that low-level exposures may have some long-term consequences.

Recommendation: Research on the toxicology of low-level, long-term exposures to chemical and biological agents and other potentially harmful agents (e.g., environmental and occupational contaminants and toxic industrial chemicals) should be continued and expanded.

Unfortunately, modeling and simulation can only partly compensate for the lack of data based on actual experiments. Evidence has shown that modeling and simulation of the performance of CB protective equipment have not been very effective.

Recommendation: The use of simulants, data from animal models, and data on human exposure should be reevaluated as part of the development of a coherent research program to determine the physiological effects of both high-level and low-level long-term exposures to chemical and biological agents. The data should then be used to determine risks and challenges.

Training for CB operations has been very inconsistent, both within and among the services.

Recommendation: Required levels of training (with the appropriate level of funding for training devices and simultants) should be established and monitored for effective unit performance throughout the services. Objective criteria should be established for determining whether current service-specific training requirements are being met.

APPENDIX E

Strategies to Protect the Health of Deployed U.S. Forces: Medical Surveillance, Record Keeping and Risk Reduction—Executive Summary

Nine years after Operations Desert Shield and Desert Storm (the Gulf War) ended in June 1991, uncertainty and questions remain about illnesses reported in a substantial percentage of the 697,000 service members who were deployed. Even though it was a short conflict with very few battle casualties or immediately recognized disease or non-battle injuries, the events of the Gulf War and the experiences of the ensuing years have made clear many potentially instructive aspects of the deployment and its hazards. Since the Gulf War, several other large deployments have also occurred, including deployments to Haiti and Somalia. Major deployments to Bosnia, Southwest Asia, and, most recently, Kosovo, are ongoing as this report is written. This report draws on lessons learned from some of these deployments to consider strategies to protect the health of troops in future deployments.

In the spring of 1996, Deputy Secretary of Defense John White met with leadership of the National Research Council and the Institute of Medicine to explore the prospect of an independent, proactive effort to learn from lessons of the Gulf War and to develop a strategy to better protect the health of troops in future deployments.

The study presented in this report developed from those discussions. The U.S. Department of Defense (DoD) sought an independent, external, and unbiased evaluation of its efforts regarding the protection of U.S. forces in four areas: (1) assessment of health risks during deployments in hostile environments, (2) technologies and methods for detection and tracking of exposures to a subset of harmful agents, (3) physical protection and decontamination, and (4) medical protection, health consequences and treatment, and medical record keeping. Studies that have addressed topics 1, 2, and 3 have been carried out concurrently by the Commission on Life Sciences and the Commission on Engineering and Technical Systems of the National Research Council.

The study presented here, carried out with staff support from the Medical Follow-up Agency of the Institute of Medicine, addresses the topics of medical protection, health consequences and treatment, and medical record keeping. The study team was charged with addressing the following:

- Prevention of adverse health outcomes that could result from exposures to threats and risks including chemical warfare and biological warfare, infectious disease, psychological stress, heat and cold injuries, unintentional injuries;
- Requirements for compliance with active duty retention standards;
- Predeployment screening, physical evaluation, and risk education for troops and medical personnel;
- Vaccines and other prophylactic agents;
- Improvements in risk communication with military personnel in order to minimize stress casualties among exposed or potentially exposed personnel;
- Improvements in the reintegration of all troops to the home environment;
- Treatment of the health consequences of prevention failures, including battle injuries, disease and non-battle injury (DNBI), acute management, and long-term follow-up;
- Surveillance for short- and long-term outcomes, to include adverse reproductive outcomes; and
- Improvement in keeping medical records, perhaps using entirely new technology, in documenting exposures, treatment, tracking of individuals through the medical evacuation system, and health/administrative outcomes. (Statement of Task, Appendix B)

Within the breadth of this charge, the study team chose to emphasize areas in which greatest needs were evident from the lessons learned from the Gulf War and other recent deployments and to treat other areas (those areas where the study team believed that it had little to offer the military) less thoroughly. Since an important motivating force for the study was the health and reproductive concerns of veterans after the Gulf War, the study team chose to focus on the major challenges for prevention and data needs indicated by the health problems widely reported by deployed forces after the Gulf War and the efforts to better understand them.

What were the lessons of the Gulf War? Briefly, one of the lessons was that even in the absence of widespread acute casualties from battle, war takes its toll on human health and well-being long after the shooting or bombing stops. Although military preventive medicine programs have developed reasonably effective countermeasures against many of the discrete disease and non-battle injury hazards of deployment, they have not yet systematically addressed the medically unexplained symptoms seen not only after the Gulf War but also after major wars dating back at least to the Civil War. The health problems reported by veterans after the Gulf War also brought out two other major and interrelated needs for improvements in preventive care for deployed forces. One is for a health surveillance system with documentation so that health events in the field are noted and responded to. Closely allied is the need for an automated medical record that can provide information about a service member's health events over his or her service career and into civilian life after military service. These three topics of medically unexplained symptoms, medical surveillance, and medical record keeping form the critical areas of emphasis of the report.

Although the study team considered the service member's life cycle of recruitment, predeployment, deployment, and postdeployment to include separation from the service, the postdeployment period appeared to be a time when, in particular, additional effort could be crucial in attending to the health of the deployed forces. The report discusses needs and opportunities for improved surveillance, special focused health care, and assistance with reintegration into the home environment during this time.

Two other major issues emerged as the study group went about its work. One serious challenge to the protection of deployed U.S. forces is that of providing the National Guard and Reserve components with the preparation and health surveillance afforded the active-duty component. The reserves play an increasingly important role in military deployments. Yet, their lack of access to the military health care system while they are inactive places serious limitations on the routine health care that they receive and the ability to monitor their health status over both the short and long term after a deployment. This problem for the reserves highlights a challenge for many active-duty service members after they separate from military service. To the extent that they receive their health care in the civilian sector and not through the U.S. Department of Veterans Affairs (VA), the capture of any data on their health care is problematic, as is the concept of a true lifetime medical record as promised by President Clinton in 1997 (White House, 1997).

A second issue that the study team came to recognize as a serious concern was that although there have been encouraging changes in DoD policy with new emphasis on what is termed Force Health Protection, these changes have not yet been reflected in the structural and cultural changes that will be needed within the services and DoD so that they may carry out the laudable new policies. Effective application of an improved health surveillance system and an integrated computer-based patient record will require concerted leadership and coordination to prevent the inexorable tendency toward "stovepiping"—that is, the development or continuation of an array of independent task- or service-specific systems that cannot meet the current needs for information exchange and follow-up.

High-level leadership and coordination are also needed to effect changes in the way in which medically unexplained symptoms are addressed in military populations. Although the problem is not unique to the military, it is regularly seen in populations who have participated in major deployments and will likely be observed after future deployments. Efforts to intervene to try to prevent or ameliorate medically unexplained symptoms are needed, as are careful evaluations of these efforts and a related research program.

Need for additional high-level leadership and coordination for military public health and preventive medicine run counter to current momentum within DoD. The medical structure of DoD is focused on the delivery of health care and the operation of the Tri-Care program (the military health maintenance organization). The costs of the health care delivery system are enormous, and management of the health care delivery system has come to dominate the DoD's medical leadership. High-quality health care is crucial to recruitment and retention of good service members, but in the current environment, the practice of military preventive medicine and military medicine appears to compete very poorly for personnel, funding, and leadership resources.

Nevertheless, DoD has made considerable efforts in several areas relevant to this study since the Gulf War. An important step occurred in November 1998, when the National Science and Technology Council (NSTC) released a plan in response to a Presidential Review Directive (National Science and Technology Council, 1998). Developed by an interagency task force with representatives from DoD, VA, and the U.S. Department of Health and Human Services (DHHS), the plan is entitled, *A National Obligation: Planning for Health Preparedness for and Readjustment of the Military, Veterans, and Their Families after Future Deployments*. The plan describes many laudable goals related to health during deployments, record keeping, research, and health risk communication that the government should implement to better safeguard military forces. Taking those efforts into account, with this report the study team proposes additional and complementary strategies to more effectively address medically unexplained symptoms, medical surveillance, and medical record keeping for future deployments, as well as other aspects of prevention such as risk communication and reintegration. The report emphasizes the need to extend medical surveillance and record keeping and other protections to the reserve components.

MEDICALLY UNEXPLAINED SYMPTOMS

Medically unexplained symptoms is the term used in this report to refer to symptoms that are not clinically explained by a medical etiology and that lead to use of the health care system. They are increasingly recognized as prevalent and persistent problems among civilian populations, in which they are associated with high levels of subjective distress and functional impairment with extensive use of health care services (Hyams, 1998; Engel and Katon, 1999). In military populations, similar medically unexplained symptom-based conditions have been observed after military conflicts dating back to the Civil War (Hyams et al., 1996) and are anticipated after future deployments (Presidential Advisory Committee on Gulf War Veterans' Illnesses, 1996b).

Clinicians and other persons working in medical surveillance must recognize that medically unexplained symptoms are just that; namely, there are no current explanations for them. Therefore, communicating the limits of modern medicine coupled with a compassionate approach to patients with medically unexplained symptoms is essential to the management of such patients. Until clear etiological factors are identified, the health care professional relies upon a body of knowledge about the management of these symptoms that has proven to be effective in many cases. Although a program of primary prevention is not feasible given the current state of knowledge, enough is known to recommend the implementation of a secondary prevention strategy. Good clinical evidence indicates that medically unexplained symptoms are much harder to treat and ameliorate once they have become chronic. It is thus important to identify the patient with medically unexplained symptoms early, when there may be a greater opportunity to restore the patient to his or her previous level of function. Providers with the clinical skills needed for medical management of these patients can then work with them toward a mutually agreed upon set of therapeutic goals that include striving to cope with residual symptoms and rehabilitation in the absence of a definitive diagnosis.

Recommendations[1]

The study team recommends that the U.S. Department of Defense develop an improved strategy to address medically unexplained symptoms, involving education, detection, evaluation, mitigation, and research. (Recommendation 6-9.[2])

- **Undertake a program of continuing education for military primary care providers to improve their clinical ability to diagnose, treat, and communicate with patients with medically unexplained symptoms. Incorporate the topic into the curricula of military graduate medical education programs such as the Uniformed Services University of the Health Sciences and the service schools for medical personnel. To the extent possible, make information about medically unexplained symptoms available and accessible to**

---

[1] Because of the large number of recommendations in this report, a subset are presented in this Executive Summary.

[2] Recommendation 6-9 is Recommendation 9 in Chapter 6.

service members and to civilian health care providers for members of the reserves.
- Carry out a pilot program to identify service members in the early stages of development of medically unexplained symptoms through the use of routinely administered self-report questionnaires (examples are noted in Chapter 6) and through informed primary care providers.
- Evaluate the efficacy of the pilot secondary prevention and treatment program, including the ability of screening questionnaires to detect early stages of medically unexplained symptoms.
- Treat medically unexplained symptoms in the primary care setting whenever possible, with referral to more intensive programs as necessary.
- Carry out a research program with prospective studies to assess the role of predisposing, precipitating, and perpetuating factors in medically unexplained symptoms. As feasible, involve academic health centers in the research efforts.

MEDICAL SURVEILLANCE

The military has launched many medical or health surveillance initiatives in the last several years in response to the problems highlighted by the Gulf War illnesses. Pre- and postdeployment questionnaires and blood draws, periodic health assessments, baseline health surveys for recruits, and improved systems for the tracking of inpatient and ambulatory care visits during deployments have all been planned or implemented to various degrees.

The multiplicity of medical surveillance-related tools that have developed reflects a genuine effort on the part of DoD and the individual services to better track and document the health of deployed forces. However, with no central authority for military public health, the tools lack coordination as part of an overall plan for achieving public health goals.

Recommendation

Clarify leadership authority and accountability for coordination of preventive medicine and environmental and health surveillance across the U.S. Department of Defense and the individual services. (Recommendation 4-16.)

Part of the work of such a body would be to coordinate and potentially consolidate the surveillance tools referred to above, such as the Recruit Assessment Program to gather baseline data from incoming recruits, the Health Evaluation and Assessment Review (HEAR) and other sources of pre- and postdeployment self-reported health status data, surveillance systems for use during deployments, exposure assessment and environmental surveillance measures, and laboratory-based surveillance. Since these tools and systems were developed independently, they do not necessarily work toward shared purposes. The study team makes the following recommendations in considering these surveillance tools as part of an armamentarium of surveillance means.

Recommendations
(additional recommendations are in Chapter 4)

- **The Recruit Assessment Program should be implemented to collect baseline health data from all recruits (active-duty, National Guard, and Reserve), and should be periodically reassessed and revised in light of its goals. Its data should be used prospectively to test hypotheses about predisposing factors for the development of disease, injury, and medically unexplained symptoms.** (Recommendation 4-1.)

- **Annually administer an improved Health Evaluation and Assessment Review (HEAR) to reserve as well as to active-duty personnel to obtain baseline health information. Refine the Health Evaluation and Assessment Review by drawing on additional survey instrument and subject matter expertise.** (See full Recommendations 4-2a and 4-2b.)

- **Reinforce the laboratory capability for public health surveillance within the military. Mandate central reporting of laboratory findings of reportable conditions.** Continue to provide increased resources to overseas laboratories for surveillance in regions of military interest. (See full Recommendation 4-6.)

- **Discontinue pre- and postdeployment health (versus readiness) questionnaires unless they are warranted for military reasons other than gathering baseline and postdeployment health status information.** (See full Recommendation 4-7.)

- **As quickly as possible, implement a deployment disease and non-battle injury surveillance system that is integrated with the patient care information system and that automatically reports information to a central medical command.** Continue efforts to capture data at the individual level as well as at aggregate levels during deployments. (See full Recommendation 4-8.)

- **Integrate the efforts of environmental surveillance, preventive medicine, clinical, and information technology personnel to ensure the inclusion of medically relevant environmental and other exposures in the individual medical record.** (Recommendation 4-9.)

Given the experiences after the Vietnam and Gulf wars, the postdeployment period is crucial for carrying out medical surveillance and providing appropriate care for returning service members. The Veterans Benefits Improvement Act of 1998 (P.L. 105-368) provides that service members will be eligible for medical care for a period of 2 years after their return from service in a theater of combat operations during a period of war or hostilities. The provision of this care without the need for establishing service-connection provides a valuable opportunity to ascertain the health needs of this population, including those related to medically unexplained symptoms. Rather than naming a special deployment-specific registry, veterans should be able to receive care as needed from the designated sources. It will be important to determine who uses this care and how well data surrounding this care can be captured from DoD and VA providers and their contractors. To gather postdeployment health status information from a more representative sample of veterans after deployments, a self-report survey could be used.

Recommendations

Carry out studies to evaluate the data captured from the 2 years of care provided after a deployment. Try to determine the extent to which the data are representative of the population of service members who deployed and whether they could be used to indicate the health of service members after a deployment. (Recommendation 4-10.)

- **Annually administer Health Evaluation and Assessment Review (HEAR) to a representative sample of service members who have been separated from the service for 2 to 5 years after a major deployment to track health status and identify health concerns including medically unexplained symptoms.** Also administer the HEAR to those separated service members who seek health care during the 2 years after a deployment. Evaluate the validity and usefulness of the information collected. (Recommendation 4-11.)
- **Avoid whenever possible the creation of deployment-specific registries. Depend, instead, on the data provided by routine medical care under the Veterans Benefits Improvement Act of 1998 (P.L. 105-368) and the annual Health Evaluation and Assessment Review.** (Recommendation 4-12.)

POSTDEPLOYMENT REINTEGRATION

The changing demographics of deployed forces, increased operational tempo, and increased reliance on the reserve component bring heightened needs for support services for service members and their families both during and after deployments. It is crucial that service members returning from deployments have seamless access to health care and support services and be made aware of the resources available to them. Since the Gulf War, the service components have made progress in providing support services to service members and families during reintegration, but the programs have not been adequately evaluated.

Recommendations

- **Planning and operational documents for military deployments should be required to include plans for supporting the return and reintegration of active-duty and reserve service members involved in the deployment and should specify the strategies that should be used to address anticipated problems, the resources needed to carry them out, and proposals for how the resources will be made available.** (See full Recommendation 7-1.)
- **Carry out research into the needs of service members and their families during deployments and upon reintegration into the home environment. Use the findings to reevaluate programs and policies.** (See full Recommendation 7-3.)

MEDICAL RECORD KEEPING

Previous studies have cited deficiencies in medical record keeping as a major impediment to understanding and treating the health effects associated with deployment to the Gulf War (Institute of Medicine, 1996a; Presidential Advisory Committee on Gulf War Veterans' Illnesses, 1996b). The study team and other health information experts consider the computer-based patient record essential for DoD to meet the health care needs of service members before, during, and after deployments. In 1996, the Presidential Advisory Committee on Gulf War Veterans' Illnesses directed the NSTC to develop an interagency plan to address health preparedness for and readjustment of veterans and families after future conflicts and peacekeeping missions (Presidential Advisory Committee on Gulf War Veterans' Illnesses, 1996b). NSTC subsequently recommended that DoD "implement a fully integrated computer-based patient record available across the entire spectrum of health care delivery over the lifetime of the patient" (National Science and Technology Council, 1998, p. 23). To serve the military health system needs, the computer-based patient record (CPR) system must meet several needs simultaneously:

1. provide access to an individual's health data anytime and anywhere that care is required,
2. support record keeping for the administration of preventive health services,

3. facilitate real-time medical surveillance of deployed forces and timely medical surveillance of the total force,

4. provide comprehensive databases that support outcomes studies and epidemiological studies, and

5. maintain longitudinal health records of service members beginning with recruitment and extending past the time of discharge from the military.

During the course of the study, the team heard briefings on several military health information system projects. In general, each need for health data has been addressed by a separate data-gathering activity at the individual service level. No central oversight authority common to all three services was apparent to ensure that independent efforts are coordinated or, better yet, consolidated into a single activity that serves the needs of all three services. The military health system has adopted a "best of breed" approach, in which task-specific software applications are interfaced together. This strategy takes advantage of multiple niche products, but it presents a significant challenge to the integration of data because of the lack of a common data model or a common database. To the extent possible, the needs of all three services should be considered concurrently to maximize the reuse of data and software programs.

In addition to the development of technical plans for data integration, organizational plans need to be developed to standardize policies and practices related to medical record keeping. Currently, guidelines for medical record documentation vary on the basis of the type of data involved (e.g., outpatient, inpatient, and immunization information), the location of the service member (e.g., garrison, deployed, and location of deployment), and the branch of service. Policies, procedures, and practices should be standardized to store consistent and comprehensive data in the computer-based patient record (CPR) throughout the military.

Recommendations
(additional recommendations are in Chapter 5)

- **Clarify leadership authority and accountability for establishment of an integrated approach to the development, implementation, and evaluation of information system applications across the military services. Establish a top-level technical oversight committee responsible for approving all architectural decisions and ensuring that all application component selections meet architecture and data standards requirements.** (Recommendation 5-1.)

- **Coordinate the evaluation of information needs for maximum reuse of data elements, data-gathering instruments (e.g., surveys), and software systems across the military health system.** (See full Recommendation 5-2.)

- **Develop standard enterprisewide policies and procedures for comprehensive medical record keeping that support the information needs of those involved with individual care, medical surveillance, and epidemiologic studies.** (Recommendation 5-3.)
- **Develop methods to gather and analyze retrievable, electronically stored health data on reservists.** (See full Recommendation 5-6.)

There are many challenges to the development, implementation, and maintenance of a health information system to serve the diverse needs of the military. It is not surprising that there are separate activities in each of the services. In some cases these separate activities are driven by immediate needs, and in other cases they arise out of a lack of awareness of existing solutions or projects under way elsewhere. To meet the needs of U.S. forces deployed abroad, however, a unified CPR system is essential. The study team recommends that a comprehensive review of the military health information systems strategy be undertaken to enumerate the information needs; define an expedient process for development of an enterprisewide technical architecture, common data model, and data standards; identify critical dependencies; establish realistic time lines; assess the adequacy of resources; and perform a realistic risk assessment with contingency plans.

The process of developing an integrated CPR for the military health care system is complex yet essential to ensuring military readiness and a healthy force. It involves a tremendous expenditure of money and resources and requires extensive expertise. With so much at stake, the study team recommends that an external advisory board participate in the effort by providing ongoing review and advice regarding the military health information systems strategy. Composed of members of academia and industry, this group would provide synergy and potential leverage between the military and civilian sectors in information systems. The study team believes that this partnership will increase the likelihood of success of the overall endeavor.

Recommendations

Conduct an independent risk assessment of the military health information systems strategy and implementation plan. Establish an external advisory board that reports to the Secretary of Defense and that is composed of members of academia, industry, and government organizations other than the Department of Defense and the Department of Veterans Affairs to provide ongoing review and advice regarding the military health information system's strategy and implementation. (Recommendation 5-4.)

Given the mandatory nature of medical data collection in the military, including sensitive information (e.g., human immunodeficiency virus infection status and mental health status), stringent regulations, policies, and procedures are necessary to maintain system security and protect the confidential medical information of all service members and their dependents.

Recommendation

Make available to service members the regulations, policies, and procedures regarding system security and protection of individually identifiable health information for each service member. (See full Recommendation 5-7.)

RISK COMMUNICATION

Risk communication has come to describe a process of concerted information and opinion exchange among individuals, groups, and institutions (National Research Council, 1989). The study team believes that a clear commitment to improvements in risk communication is needed from DoD. Responsibility should be designated to attempt a change in the culture within DoD and the military services so that dialogue and exchange about risks are facilitated at all levels. Aspects of risk communication need to be incorporated into the training programs for line commanders and health care providers. Furthermore, discussion is needed within DoD and the services about what problems the tool of risk communication may be used to try to solve. Such a discussion can lead to goals for reducing those problems and means of evaluation and improvement.

The risk communication efforts associated with the vaccination against anthrax, the risk communication goal articulated in Presidential Review Directive 5, the guide developed in response to recommendations from earlier independent advisory bodies, and the *Comprehensive Risk Communication Plan for Gulf War Veterans* (Persian Gulf Veterans Coordinating Board, 1999) are encouraging signs that the importance of risk communication has been acknowledged within some quarters at DoD. An additional indication of commitment to a cultural change throughout the entire system is needed from the top.

Recommendation

Although responsibility for risk communication must permeate all levels of command, the U.S. Department of Defense (DoD) should designate and provide resources to a group within DoD that is given primary responsibility for developing and implementing a plan to achieve the risk communication goal articulated in the Na-

tional Science and Technology Council's Presidential Review Directive 5. (Recommendation 6-1.) **Such a plan should**

- Involve service members, their families, and outside experts in developing an explicit set of risk communication topics and goals. In other words, decide what information people need to know and when they need to know it.
- Consider how to deliver the information, including the intensity of communication needed for different types of risks. Some topics will necessitate full, ongoing dialogue between the involved parties, whereas others will require less extensive efforts. Incorporate procedures to evaluate the success of risk communication efforts and use these evaluations to revise the communication plan as needed.
- Include a response plan to anticipate the inevitable appearance of new risks or health concerns among deployed forces. The plan should include a process for gathering and disseminating information (both about the risks themselves and about the concerns of the troops) and for evaluating how communications about these issues are received and understood by service members and their families.
- Educate communicators, including line officers and physicians, in relevant aspects of risk communication.
- Carry out the interagency applied research program described in Presidential Review Directive 5, Strategy 5.1.2.

RESERVES

Several of the most important components of a strategy to protect the health of deployed forces (improved medical surveillance and care that is responsive to medically unexplained symptoms, record keeping, risk communication, the use of preventive measures, and reintegration into the home environment) pose particular challenges for the reserve component because of their quasicivilian status and geographically dispersed situation. Since the Ready Reserve now constitutes almost half of the total force and is a significant component of deployed forces, the needs of the reserves cannot be ignored or postponed. Although their special circumstances make it impossible to mandate a health protection strategy identical to that for the active-duty forces, a coherent strategy should be developed to provide similar programs working toward the same ends that are provided with adequate resources.

Recommendation

Include the reserves in the planning, coordination, and implementation of improved health surveillance, record keeping, and risk communication. Develop a strategy for the reserve forces that takes into consideration their limited access to the military health care system before and after deployments but that recognizes their particular needs for health protection and that provides adequate resources to meet those needs. (See full Recommendation 8-1.)

CONCLUSIONS

Since the Gulf War, DoD has demonstrated much greater awareness of the importance of medical surveillance and record keeping in protecting the health of its deployed forces. It has launched or planned a variety of initiatives to address acknowledged shortcomings in these areas. These efforts suffer from a lack of the concerted planning required for efficient use of systems and resources. For medical surveillance this might be addressed with leadership and coordination in the area of military public health. With medical record keeping, outside expert review is needed to provide ongoing input into the challenging effort of implementing a successful CPR for the military.

The medically unexplained symptoms reported by veterans after the Gulf War have motivated many of DoD's constructive changes in medical surveillance and medical record keeping, but these initiatives cannot be anticipated to prevent them after future deployments. Indeed, it is not yet known how medically unexplained symptoms can be prevented. Better medical surveillance and record keeping can lay the foundation so that similar questions can be more readily answered in the future, however, and permit better insights into questions of etiology. The study team urges a research effort to obtain a better understanding of predisposing, precipitating, and perpetuating factors for these conditions. In the meantime, steps should be taken to identify those suffering from medically unexplained symptoms and intervene with management and treatment of symptoms to mitigate them and prevent chronicity. The efficacies of these steps should be evaluated.

APPENDIX F

Acknowledgments

The study team is grateful to the following individuals who provided information and assistance to the project through presentations at meetings and workshops, technical review, or other means.

MAJ Jeffrey Adamovicz
520th Theater Area Medical Lab

CAPT Lawrence Betts
Navy Environmental Health Center

Col Dana Bradshaw
Air Force Medical Operations Agency

Dr. Mark Brown
U.S. Department of Veterans Affairs

LtCol Steve Channel
Wright Patterson Air Force Base

RADM Cowan
Office of the Assistant Secretary of Defense for Health Affairs

COL Robert DeFraites
U.S. Army Center for Health Promotion and Preventive Medicine

LTC Charles Engel Jr., MD, MPH
Walter Reed Army Medical Center
Uniformed Services University of the Health Sciences

MG (ret) George Friel
Formerly of U.S. Army Soldier and Biological Chemical Command

Dr. Henry Gardner
U.S. Army Center for Environmental Health Research

Col John Graham
British Liaison Office

Dr. Jack Heller
U.S. Army Center for Health Promotion and Preventive Medicine

COL Ken Hoffman
Military and Veterans Health Coordinating Board

CAPT Craig Hyams
Naval Medical Research Center

LtCol Larry Kimm
Medical Readiness Division, J-4

BGen Richard Lynch MC
U.S. Army Reserve
Commander, 332nd Medical Brigade

Major Mike Malone, USMC
U.S. Joint Forces Command

RADM Mayo
Medical Readiness Division, J-4

CAPT Wayne McBride
Navy Bureau of Medicine and Surgery

Dr. Enrique Mendez
Former Assistant Secretary of Defense for Health Affairs

LTC Jane Meyer
Office of the Assistant Secretary of Defense for Health Affairs

LtCol Mary Ann Morreale, USAF
Health Care Reengineering
TriCare Management Activity

Mr. Mike Parker
U.S. Army Soldier and Biological Chemical Command

SCPO James Piner
Armed Forces Medical Intelligence Center

Mr. Tom Pease
Gentex Corporation

Col Craig Postelwaite
Military and Veterans Health Coordinating Board

Mr. John Resta
U.S. Army Center for Health Promotion and Preventive Medicine

Dr. Roy Reuter
Life Systems, Inc.

LtCol James Riddle
Office of the Assistant Secretary of Defense for Health Affairs

LTC Mark Rubertone
U.S. Army Center for Health Promotion and Preventive Medicine

Major Bruce Ruscio
Office of the Undersecretary of Defense for Environmental Security

LTC Robert Thompson
Office of the Assistant Secretary of Defense for Health Affairs

CAPT Dave Trump
Office of the Assistant Secretary of Defense for Health Affairs

Dr. John Weimaster
U.S. Army Soldier and Biological Chemical Command

Dr. Eugene Wilusz
Natick Soldier Center

Dr. Ngai Wong
U.S. Army Soldier and Biological
  Chemical Command

Special thanks are extended to the principal investigators of the four reports completed in the first 2 years of this project:

Dr. Lorenz Rhomberg
Gradient Corporation

Dr. Michael Wartell
Indiana University

Dr. Thomas McKone
School of Public Health
University of California at Berkeley

Dr. Samuel Guze (deceased)
Washington University School of
  Medicine

Dr. Michael Kleinman
University of California at Irvine

Dr. Philip Russell
Johns Hopkins School of Hygiene
  and Public Health

APPENDIX G

Committee Biographies

JOHN H. MOXLEY III, M.D. (*Chair*), is the Managing Director of the North American Health Care Division, and a partner of the Physician Executive Practice of Korn/Ferry International. His Academy experience includes membership in the Institute of Medicine, the Information Panel of the Council on Health Care Technology, the COSEPUP Panel on Ensuring the Best Science and Technology Presidential Appointments, and the Board on Army Science and Technology. He is a director of the Henry M. Jackson Foundation for the Advancement of Military Medicine and formerly the Assistant Secretary of Defense for Health Affairs. He held deanships at the University of Maryland and the University of California, San Diego, medical schools. He is board certified in Internal Medicine and a Fellow of the American College of Physicians.

RUTH L. BERKELMAN, M.D., is currently with the Rollins School of Public Health, Emory University. An Assistant Surgeon General, she has served as a Senior Adviser to the Director, Centers for Disease Control and Prevention (CDC) and is a member of the Board of Trustees of Princeton University. She was formerly the deputy director of the National Center for Infectious Diseases and led CDC's efforts to respond to the threat of emerging infectious diseases. Board certified in pediatrics and internal medicine, she also serves on the American Society of Microbiology's Committee on Public Health and is a member of the American Epidemiological Society and a Fellow of the Infectious Diseases Society of America. She has extensive experience in disease surveillance and is a member of the Institute of Medicine Committee to Review the

DoD Global Emerging Infections Surveillance and Response System (DoD-GEIS) Strategic Plan.

J. CRIS BISGARD, M.D., M.P.H., has been the Director of Health Services at Delta Air Lines, Inc. since 1994. Previously, he was the Corporate Medical Director at Pacific Bell. Dr. Bisgard was a member of the U.S. Air Force until he retired after 23 years with the rank of Colonel. He served as the acting Deputy Assistant Secretary of Defense (Health Affairs) for 3 years. He is a fellow of the Aerospace Medicine Association, the American College of Preventive Medicine, and the American College of Physician Executives. Dr. Bisgard serves on the Board of Directors at Trilinear, Inc., the Washington Business Group on Health, and the Epidermolysis Bullosa Medical Research Foundation (EBMRF). He is also a member of the International Academy of Aviation and Space Medicine. Dr. Bisgard previously served on the Institute of Medicine Committee to Review the Breast Cancer Research Program.

GUY LABOA is currently employed by CIBA Vision as Executive Director of Dailies Manufacturing. Prior to his employment at CIBA Vision he served in the U.S. Army for 35 years and retired as a Lieutenant General in 1997. During his senior executive service in the military, he commanded the First United States Army, served as chief of staff of the United States Forces Command, and commanded the 4th Infantry Division (Mech.) at Fort Carson, among numerous senior posts. His awards include the Distinguished Service Medal, the Silver Star, the Legion of Merit, and the Purple Heart.

LAYTON McCURDY, M.D., is the Vice President for Medical Affairs, Dean of the College of Medicine, and Professor of Psychiatry at the Medical University of South Carolina. Dr. McCurdy has made contributions to the scientific literature in the areas of medical education, addiction, psychopharmacology, and current issues in psychiatry. He served as Chair of the American Psychiatric Association's Committee on Psychiatric Diagnosis and Assessment.

MATTHEW L. PUGLISI is currently employed as the Government Relations Manager for the Optical Society of America, an association of optical scientists involved with technologies to include fiber optics and lasers. Prior to his employment with OSA he was employed with the American Legion representing Gulf War veterans' interests before the federal government. He served on the Department of Veterans Affairs Gulf War Expert Scientific Committee. Mr. Puglisi served in the Persian Gulf with the U.S. Marines during Operation Desert Shield/Desert Storm, and is currently a Major in the Marine Reserves.

LYNN A. STREETER, Ph.D., is currently working as a consultant for Knowledge Analysis Technologies, LLC. Dr. Streeter has extensive experience in the

Information Management sector, highlighted by her work managing a large software R&D organization for many years at U.S. West, as well as previously directing computer science- and behavioral science-related groups at Bellcore and Bell Laboratories. Her Academy experience includes authoring a report for the National Research Council's Committee on Future Technologies for Army Multimedia Communications.

ELAINE VAUGHAN, Ph.D., is Associate Professor in the Department of Psychology and Social Behavior at the School of Social Ecology of the University of California, Irvine. Her research interests and expertise are in risk communication, management, and the public's evaluation of and response to technological, medical, and environmental risks. Dr. Vaughan has served on California's Committee on Comparative Risk Policy and the University of California's Scientific Advisory Panel on Low-Level Radioactive Waste Disposal, and previously served on the National Research Council Committee on Risk Characterization.

LAUREN ZEISE, Ph.D., is Chief of the Reproductive and Cancer Hazard Assessment Section within the Office of Environmental Health Hazard Assessment, California Environmental Protection Agency. Her research interests and expertise are in risk assessment and risk modeling. She has served on several National Research Council and Institute of Medicine committees including the Committee on Risk Characterization and the Committee on Assessment of Wartime Exposure to Herbicides in Vietnam.